Suffering in Theology and Medical Ethics

Christof Mandry (Ed.)

Suffering in Theology and Medical Ethics

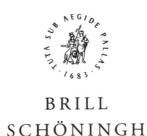

BRILL
SCHÖNINGH

Bibliographic information published by the Deutsche Nationalbibliothek

The Deutsche Nationalbibliothek lists this publication in the Deutsche Nationalbibliografie; detailed bibliographic data available online: http://dnb.d-nb.de

© 2022 by Brill Schöningh, Wollmarktstraße 115, 33098 Paderborn, Germany, an imprint of the Brill-Group (Koninklijke Brill NV, Leiden, The Netherlands; Brill USA Inc., Boston MA, USA; Brill Asia Pte Ltd, Singapore; Brill Deutschland GmbH, Paderborn, Germany; Brill Österreich GmbH, Vienna, Austria) Koninklijke Brill NV incorporates the imprints Brill, Brill Nijhoff, Brill Hotei, Brill Schöningh, Brill Fink, Brill mentis, Vandenhoeck & Ruprecht, Böhlau, Verlag Antike and V&R unipress.

www.schoeningh.de

Cover design: Anna Braungart, Tübingen
Production: Brill Deutschland GmbH, Paderborn

ISBN 978-3-506-71542-5 (paperback)
ISBN 978-3-657-71542-8 (e-book)

Contents

Human Suffering at the Shared Interface of Medicine, Philosophy
and Theology: Introduction IX
    Christof Mandry

PART I
People Suffering: Philosophical, Theological and Medical Approaches

1   **Pain and the Human Condition** 3
    Arne Johan Vetlesen

2   **"... somewhere very close to me ..." – Aspects of an Anthropology
of Suffering: The Transformative Passivity of Aesthetic
Experience** 13
    Knut Wenzel

3   **The Concept of Suffering in the Context of Palliative Medicine** ... 30
    Bernd Oliver Maier

4   **Suffering in the Context of Mental Illness: A Challenge for
Ethics in Psychiatry** 41
    Gwendolin Wanderer

PART II
Suffering in the Medical-Ethical Discourse: An Uncomfortable Concept

5   **The Argument of "Suffering" in Opinions of the German Ethics
Council (2007-2016)** 61
    Michael Coors

6   **Suffering – an Increasingly Relevant, Though Ambivalent
Concept in Bioethics** 75
    Claudia Bozzaro

7 Suffering as Challenge for the Practice and Identity of Medicine:
The Case of *Body Integrity Identity Disorder* 86
Tobias Eichinger

8 Suffering in the Islamic Tradition and Its Meaning for Intercultural
Medical Ethics 97
Tuba Erkoc Baydar, Ilhan Ilkilic

PART III
*Broadening the View: Narrative-Ethical and Theological
Contributions*

9 Uprooted – Towards a Medical Ethics of Suffering 113
Hille Haker

10 Medical Technology and the Body: Narrative Ethics in Simone de
Beauvoir's *A Very Easy Death* 145
Tara Flanagan

11 Prenatal Genetic Testing & the Complicated Quest for a
Healthy Baby: Christian Ethics in Conversation with Genetic
Counselors 160
Aana Marie Vigen

12 Responding from the Place of Suffering: Informed Consent and
Non-invasive Prenatal Genetic Screening 179
Michael McCarthy

PART IV
Spirituality and Religion in Care and Ethical Counselling

13 Suffering in the Practice of the Christian Faith in God 191
Ottmar Fuchs

14 "Will you still need me ...?" – Health Care Chaplaincy in the
Face of Suffering 204
Jürgen Janik

15   Humanist Approaches to Spiritual Care in Patient Counseling
      in the Netherlands 214
         Carlo Leget

16   Psychological and Psychotherapeutic Counseling of Palliative
      Care Patients 226
         Urs Münch

17   Professionalizing Clinical Ethics Consultation: Training to
      Encounter Human Suffering via the Assessing Clinical Ethics
      Skills Tool 233
         Katherine Wasson

      Contributors 243

Human Suffering at the Shared Interface of Medicine, Philosophy and Theology

Introduction

Christof Mandry

People can suffer from many things – for example from loneliness, poverty, disregard, pain, hopelessness, the loss of a loved one, from unrequited love or the prospect of having to die. It is therefore unsurprising that human suffering is one of the major topics in arts, literature and religion, on a par and interwoven with other major human issues such as love and the pursuit of peace and justice.

What is suffering? Suffering is obviously a conscious feeling, since certain situations alone do not cause suffering. Loneliness, for example, can be self-imposed. In certain situations, people accept suffering as an acceptable price to pay for other things: pain for success, such as in competitive sports, or other people's disregard for any other value considered worth suffering for. What to some might seem an obvious disadvantage or negative experience does not necessarily have to involve suffering: pain and disregard, while not being pleasant or positive, do not necessarily have to involve suffering. In this, the ineluctable subjectivity of suffering becomes obvious. This even applies to illness and disability which we usually associate with suffering. In learning to live with their illness, patients often do not suffer, or only rarely suffer, from the illness itself; people with disabilities often state that they do not suffer from them, but rather from the pitiful looks from their fellow human beings who regard their conditions of living as deplorable and deficient.

It therefore seems important to not just consider suffering in terms of certain incidents or situations in life which usually are associated with suffering, but to acknowledge the importance of the subjective dimension of suffering. Human beings try to find meaning in their experiences and to make sense of their life's journey Does this mean that suffering is to be interpreted as futility, as the inability even, to make sense of certain incidents, experiences or situations in life? Do people suffer from not being able to derive meaning from something, from not being able to fit it into their life story, from the inability to make sense of something and from the probability of not being able to find acceptance for this inability in other people? Or does suffering actually imply its own, different interpretation, namely that something is pointless, absurd, vain, appalling, embarrassing and degrading; and furthermore that it thereby acquires a meaning, even if this meaning is negative and often inexpressible except by outcry? An outcry to whom? To fate, silent fellow humans, one's own helplessness, an absent God?

One of the traditional tasks of Religion is to provide meaning where normal everyday life is interrupted and the typical ideas that offer orientation fail to convince. Religions offer a multitude of pictures, teachings, tales and rituals in which crises are overcome, and which have the potential to help people live through their own crises. Religions also offer practices that enable people to react empathically to crises of their fellow human beings. Practices of solidarity cannot provide meaning, but they can support living and suffering through crises. In this, they achieve more than just to endure the unendurable, for even suffering has a time-based dimension. The end of the path of suffering might yet be out of sight, but it is comforting and encouraging to know that this path must not necessarily be travelled alone. Can medicine function as such a practice of solidarity, and if so, under which conditions? What forms can supporting the sufferer and alleviating suffering take in modern societies that are based on the division of labor and pluralism?

In fact, in our societies, disease is almost invariably equated with suffering. This is what leads to medicine and health care as professional institutions almost having a social mandate to eliminate and alleviate suffering. It has been often and rightly objected that this simple equation is inaccurate and that disease is not identical with illness. This also applies the other way round: The cause of physical and mental suffering does not only and sometimes not even primarily lie in biological and physiological disorders of the body and psyche. Poverty, injustice, racial and sexual violence, social and cultural marginalization and poor environmental conditions can cause physical and mental suffering as well. Suffering caused by these factors includes illness and may materialize as illness, but it goes beyond this. The relation between disease, illness, suffering and the mission and mandate of health care professions is therefore very complex. Surprisingly, very little thought is given to suffering in medical education and medical treatment. This issue was the subject of Eric Cassel's influential essay (Cassel 1982).

Traditionally, as Cassel points out, alleviating suffering is an integral part of medicine's basic mission, but it appears that medicine's relationship to human suffering is not so clear-cut. Medical treatment can be associated with suffering, for example when causing severe side effects. The perceptions of physicians and patients can differ greatly, and what is considered a success for physicians may have little or no benefit from the patient's perspective, since, from this point of view, suffering is only deferred by the treatment. The fact that their point of view is given so little consideration can be perceived by patients as distressing. Patients often experience feelings of alienation when in hospital; they feel subordinated to the institution's procedures and hierarchies. Furthermore, the sort of disadvantage and discrimination that people are subjected to even outside the health care system and that probably lie at the roots of their illness and suffering often simply continue within medical care. Cassel hence argued in favor of focusing more on the patient's subjective feeling of suffering and thus presenting an alternative to the medical-biological disease model. Ever since, there has actually been a stronger focus on the subjective dimension of illness. Clearly, reducing the concept of illness merely to the experience of pain would mean ignoring the fact that the patient's wishes are not being taken into account; this is in fact a major cause for the suffering of patients within the medical system. Cassel eventually suggested acknowledging the endangerment of personal integrity as the root of suffering: "Most generally, suffering can be defined as the state of severe distress associated with events that threaten the intactness of the person." (Cassel 1982, p. 640)

This suggestion has started a lively and ongoing discussion about the subjective and the objective dimensions of disease, illness and sickness as well as their interrelation. Is a standardized concept of illness even possible? Perhaps as a form of self-alienation, which physicians and medical ethicists have to empathize with to do their patients justice? (Svenaeus 2018) But what is the precise meaning of the patient's physical and psychological perception in medicine and ethics, especially with regard to the difficulty of articulating it, and to its volatility? (Hauskeller 2018) The crucial significance attached to patient autonomy in clinical ethics consultation as well as in medical law adds to the complexity of the problem. Any person suffering from a disease can expect to be treated as a patient and thus generally has a moral and legal right to medical treatment. In the concept of autonomy, a moral and an epistemic aspect are closely connected in this context. The moral aspect of autonomy consists in the patient's right of decision regarding their situation and their treatment. The epistemic aspect lies in the patient's privileged access to relevant information, namely their personal experience of their illness (whether and to what extent they suffer from it) and their wishes (as to how they want to be treated and their plans for life). The patients know best what the illness means for them, how it impedes them and how having to live with a disease, its consequences or a resulting disability affects their plans for life and their self-perception. Ultimately, only the patient can tell whether they are ill at all – whether they are suffering from their physiological condition and want to appeal to others for help. This connection of moral and epistemic aspects raises important questions for medicine and ethics. Can a person err in their subjective feeling, for example when they suffer without cause, or when they do not suffer in a situation that "objectively" gives them every reason to suffer? What is the relevance of suffering when a disturbed self-perception is part of the pathology as in personality disorder traits? In this case, is suffering "from oneself" part of the cure? To what kind and what extent of medical treatment and care do patients have a moral right by virtue of their suffering and their claim to self-determination? From an equity-based point of view, must this not somehow be covered by objective, i.e. intersubjectively comprehensible, reasons? Or do ethical reasons forbid turning away suffering persons because the disregard of suffering can in itself be a cause of suffering?

Obviously, suffering poses a challenge to thinking because of its multiplicity. Human suffering cannot easily be expressed in the terminologies of medicine, philosophy and ethics. This certainly has to do with the fact that suffering initially renders people speechless. Where suffering is successfully articulated, it is often rather in a stammer, stutter and stumble than through language, verging on the incomprehensible. And how could it be otherwise? At best, and often only little by little, suffering people manage to express their suffering in metaphors, pictures, stories, maybe poetry, maybe even in language forms they have to borrow for themselves, since they otherwise would be rendered speechless. This is how religion happens, how literature functions: as safety lines for language teetering on the precipice of speechlessness. Accordingly, it cannot be the task of suffering to find its way into the terminologies of science, philosophy and theology. Instead, they have to bridge the gap towards experiences and expressions of suffering. This is what the essays in this book are trying to do in their interdisciplinary approaches, coming from medicine, philosophy, theology and ethics.

The first section, *People suffering: Philosophical, theological and medical approaches*, encompasses contributions about the phenomenon and the perception of suffering in humans.

In his philosophical essay, Arne Johan Vetlesen poses the question whether something would be missing if human existence were to be completely free of pain and suffering. He examines the tension between the negative validation of pain as something hardly desirable and the significance of sensitivity to suffering and pain in our entire culture. The fact that humans share vulnerability through pain and suffering connects them in a profound way and lies at the root of certain cultural forms of solidarity which we may not want to give up.

Through intensive dialogue with literature and poetry, Knut Wenzel makes aesthetical observations on linguistic expressions of pain and suffering. He acknowledges it as a basic dimension of human existence which, in accordance with Greek culture, he identifies as *pathos*, a fundamental passivity and susceptibility in human beings. Can an aesthetical experience be implicit even in pain and agony? Not to say that there is anything beautiful in pain or agony, but that in impact and overpowering, pain and aesthetic experience have a common dimension. In the experience of pain, so he observes, the subject also experiences itself as deeply severed, as not identical with its own existence.

Bernd Oliver Maier, a palliative physician, writes from the perspective of treating patients who have come to the end of their lives and are ravaged by disease. Palliative care has learned to pay attention to various aspects of suffering such as the physical, psychological and, last but not least, existential. In doing this, palliative care leaves it to the patient to decide which aspect of their suffering is oppresses them the most. According to Maier, in palliative care, ultimately, it comes down to having a deep respect for the individual patient so as to be able to take them seriously in their existential suffering.

The text by Gwendolin Wanderer takes up and explores the acknowledgement that suffering is essentially subjectively determined. She deliberates on the concept of mental suffering and how the suffering experiences of the mentally ill are to be considered. How can a patient's individual wishes and plans for life be honored in therapeutic decisions, if the personality of the patient is altered by their psychiatric condition? Closely oriented towards patient narratives, she explores the ambiguity and opacity of suffering.

This already touches upon ethical considerations focused on in the second section of this book, *Suffering in the medical-ethical discourse: an uncomfortable concept*. How can the significance of suffering in medical ethics possibly be defined?

In examining the statements of the German Ethics Council, Michael Coors elaborates their implicit concept of suffering. For although suffering plays a major role in public controversies about many bio-ethical and medical-ethical topics, it is actually not explicitly present in the conventional medical-ethical principles of non-maleficence, beneficence, autonomy and justice. Through a semantic analysis, Coors differentiates four manners of use of "suffering" by the German Ethics Council. One major issue is how a third party can be able to attribute suffering to a person, if that person would not or cannot express it, as is the case with unborn children or people alive in the future.

Claudia Bozzaro also refers to the categories of suffering in medical ethics. In appreciating the autonomy of the patient and in respecting the subjective view of the patient, patients' expressions of suffering also carry more moral weight. This is especially true for the category "unbearable suffering", which has been used for a while now in jurisdiction and in medical-ethical discourse, for example as an argument in the context of palliative sedation or terminal sedation. Apart from the subjective and objective concepts of suffering, Bozzaro also discusses a social concept of suffering and enquires after their validity in medical-ethical decision-making.

Tobias Eichinger deals with the extreme case of Body Integrity Identity Disorder, where people suffer from healthy and functional organs and wish for their surgical removal. Is it ethically justifiable, or even appropriate, to accept this wish, or is this wish to be rejected as objectively unreasonable, since the organ is healthy? Eichinger disputes whether following the patient's will in this case also is a natural consequence of the concept of the autonomy of the patient, or whether in this case a limit has been reached for the ethical significance of the concept of suffering.

In their essay, Tuba Erkoc Baydar and Ilhan Ilkilic point out the cultural embeddedness of concepts of suffering. They examine the Islamic discourse about existential and medical suffering and evaluate it with regard to interculturally sensitive medical ethics. Using ethical counselling on the occasion of a controversial change of the therapeutic goal as an example, they show that intercultural introspection can indeed be of benefit when it comes to grasping both the meaning of suffering as well as the patient's best interest.

The third section, *Broadening the View: Narrative-ethical and theological contributions*, further addresses the question of the embedding of medical-ethical concepts and introspections by viewing experiences of illness and medical decision-making in the context of patients' personal histories. Personal histories mirror people's experiences and sufferings in the context of social and economic coherence, of more or less equal opportunities, of the hopes and meaning (both religious and secular) people attach to their lives.

Hille Hakes refers to the passive character of suffering as affect ("Widerfahrnis") and outlines an ethic of appropriate interaction with suffering individuals in the medical context. This form of ethics applies not only to the justification of how physicians and carers act, but also to the language of health care professionals in communicating with, and their attitude towards, suffering and dying patients. In this, she strictly assumes the point of view of the patients and their relatives – the phenomenology and narrative of their experiences of suffering. Especially these narratives show that the personal histories of the patient are entangled with those of the relatives. Compassionate and consolatory attitudes, far from fostering false hopes, are rooted in the common experience of vulnerability.

Tara Flanagan also bases her essay on a narrative: Simone de Beauvoir's "A Very Easy Death", where the author describes the death of her mother. Flanagan analyzes the social and institutional patterns which de Beauvoir depicts and questions in her account of her mother's death, reflecting on the values thus literary expressed by de Beauvoir. Afterwards, Flanagan continues to describe the medicalization of death in contemporary culture and reflects on the role of the hospice movement in this context.

Aana Marie Vigen, on the contrary, discusses a very different topic, namely reproductive medicine and prenatal genetics in the United States. Through her interviews with genetic counselors, she uncovers social and societal factors that influence people's decisions to make use of prenatal genetic screening, such as ethnic and social status, existence of sufficient health care insurance, language skills and level of education. This makes obvious the sufferings of persons of color or of Latin-American descent, who, despite the principle of autonomy that applies to gynecology, are not respected as individuals.

Michael McCarthy continues to deal with this topic in the field of non-invasive prenatal screening (NIPS) and questions the generally accepted medical practice of informed consent. If informed consent for many female patients simply means having the choice of accepting or declining a certain form of treatment, then this is based on a very shallow concept of "free choice". This sort of "free choice" ignores the prerequisites and circumstances that ultimately may have led to the women's decisions, as McCarthy shows in applying the Latin-American feminist (mujerista) theory of *Lo cotidiano*. The question is: If the realities of life of the female patients are radically different from those of the health care professionals, how can a just and appropriate practice of medical counseling possibly be established?

The fourth section, *Spirituality and religion in care and ethical counselling*, focusses on counselling and consultation practice. As has already become clear, existential, spiritual and religious aspects of illness and suffering of humans are always present and demand adequate consideration. How do concepts of pastoral and ethical counselling in different professions attempt to do justice to this fact? And does the counselling of suffering persons itself have a spiritual dimension?

From a Christian theological perspective, Ottmar Fuchs develops a basic understanding of the suffering of a religious individual. It is not necessarily the case that, when suffering, religious people find an easy comfort in their faith. Rather, there is a form of religious suffering arising from absence and incomprehensibility. Fuchs utilizes the language repertoire of the Bible and thus shows how pleas, laments and thanks could be models for dealing with suffering. The biblical understanding is that suffering makes people aware of the inevitability of death, but also contains a glimmer of hope that death will be overcome.

From his experience in hospital pastoral care, Jürgen Janik writes about the polymorphism of suffering and how dealing with it poses a challenge to spiritual care. He describes the phenomenon of spiritual suffering, which may contain a religious component, but must not prematurely be interpreted in religious terms by pastoral carers. Religious and spiritual care and counselling, says Janik, is "practical ethics" and refuses a false urge for wholeness.

With a view from the Netherlands, Carlo Leget introduces a concept of non-religious, humanistic spiritual counselling. Revolving around the metaphor of the "inner space", the concept entails three key competences which he presents using the example of a new *ars moriendi*.

The range of professions that offer counselling and care in the palliative field also includes psychologists. Urs Münch presents the tasks, roles and competences of psychological palliative care and reveals its workings with the example of three psychotherapeutic intervention models.

In light of the plurality of professions involved in clinical ethical counselling, there is a growing need for available and evaluated ethics education instruments. Katherine Wasson introduces one of the first successfully established online tools for training and evaluation of ethical counselling. Since, for many patients, experiences of disregard in hospitals add to their suffering, a respectful and appropriate form of communication in ethical counselling is one of the key competences the program presented by Wasson aims to train.

I would like to express thanks to all the people who have made this volume possible: to the authors for their contributions, their trust and their cooperation; to current and former members of staff at the Chair for Moral Theology and Social Ethics, Franziska Schmitt, Carla Sicking and Lara Genath for their editorial and administrative support; and to Margarete Mandry and Selina Roßgardt for translations and linguistic corrections. I accept full responsibility for any remaining errors. I hope that this volume may find an interested readership and be able to contribute to the discourse about the meaning of human suffering in medicine, theology and ethics.

Bibliography

Cassel, Eric J. (1982): The nature of suffering and the goals of medicine. In: *The New England Journal of Medicine* 306 (11), p. 639-645.

Hauskeller, Michael (2018): Illness as a Crisis of Meaning. In: *The Hastings Center report* 48 (4), p. 42-43. DOI: 10.1002/hast.859.

Svenaeus, Fredrik (2018): Phenomenological bioethics. Medical technologies, human suffering, and the meaning of being alive. London, New York: Routledge Taylor & Francis Group.

PART I

People Suffering: Philosophical, Theological and Medical Approaches

Pain and the Human Condition

Arne Johan Vetlesen

Human existence as we know it is unthinkable without pain. With it, though, life is hardly to be endured. When pain becomes total, it deprives us of life and makes us long for the absence of pain – even though that would ultimately amount to an end to life. If life becomes only a matter of pain, the question is whether it is worth living.

To be alive involves being susceptible to pain every second – not necessarily as an insistent reality, but always as a possibility. Of course, some people experience more pain than others. But the fundamental exposure to pain is something all human beings share – it is an essential part of the human condition.

The individual's relation to pain and what it means for her cannot be exclusively determined by that individual. The epoch and culture in which we live and the society into which we are socialized equip each one of us with a specific vocabulary and yardstick for communicating about pain and assessing its significance. This vocabulary and this yardstick are both eminently contingent and liable to change, even though as members of the culture in question we may perceive them as wholly natural and as self-evidently valid. So whereas we typically take the experience of pain to be spontaneous, everything to do with what that pain means to us and how we relate to it – do we express the discomfort it causes, or do we hide or deny it? – is a matter of how our own individual history of pain (biography) is shaped by the culture we are part of. The raw, elementary or primitive phenomenological nature of pain in its bodily or sensorial form should not make us think that the way we react to, say, physically imposed pain is simple and forthright, as it were. Pain is not an objective datum, not a simple, self-identical 'in-itself', but always a 'for-itself', whereby the meaning of my personal experience of pain is shaped by socio-cultural patterns of responding to it, interpreting and assessing it. Such patterns differ between cultures and epochs; they also vary from one epoch to the next within each distinct culture, especially in times of increased societal acceleration.

While eminently phenomenologically subject-related, it does not follow that the way in which the individual in question relates to her pain is authentic. It may be the opposite, as in cases of split, of dissociation, of being so alienated from the pain suffered as to deny it any impact, any psychic reality whatsoever. Such mechanisms of splitting – "this is not happening to me"; or "this is happening to a part of me (of my body) from which I can manage to distance myself completely" – are well-known in instances of traumatic violence such

© BRILL SCHÖNINGH, 2022 | DOI:10.30965/9783657715428_002

as rape or torture; in the extreme cases, they are a strategy for sheer survival. For all that, the mechanisms are neither automatic (instinctual) nor wholly for the individual to decide; they are always culturally mediated and negotiated in the social context in which the pain is being inflicted. Moreover, the kind of relationship a victim has to her perpetrator will also influence her response, depending on whether, for example, she buys into the perpetrator's insistence that the pain is well deserved, that it matches the badness and lack of worth of her person.

To be sure, a case can be made that the meaning of pain is perfectly straight-forward: Pain is negative, unequivocally so. This at least seems to hold for cases of physical pain: My axe misses the block of wood and hits my leg instead. I immediately cry out loud. When pain is the stimulus, suffering is the response, understood as the protest made by the organism, a "no" ("go away from me") to what has been inflicted. The meaning of pain accordingly seems perfectly plain, invariably and objectively so: It is the inherent negativity of pain. As a creature with a body and senses, I am not free to determine whether pain is neg-ative or not. Pain presents itself as something that by its very nature is *against* me; therefore, my spontaneous response is to be *against* it. It has the char-acter of something that should not be, something undesirable by definition. Pain represents my enemy, something opposing – threatening, undermining – everything I desire, indeed, ultimately, my capacity to be *someone* who actively and energetically desires anything at all, sets goals and pursues projects in the world – so how can I not prefer the absence of pain when compared with its presence? Thus, I oppose it. Being non-neutral in this respect, the human manner of relating to the reality of pain seems to be intrinsically asymmetric: Where there is a natural tendency to seek its absence, the onus of proof is on those who would deem its presence desirable. Approving of pain rather than disapproving of it is conspicuous and prompts the need for explanation and justification, the nature of which will of course depend on whether the pain considered desirable is inflicted on others or on oneself. Deliberately hurting others is something we are culturally prepared to morally condemn; the case of deliberately harming oneself is more complicated, both psychologically and morally, inviting questions about pathology.

But then again, it is not that simple. That the meaning of pain should be tan-tamount to our wishing its disappearance from life as we live it is in itself the expression of a view that to a high degree is historically and culturally deter-mined. Indeed, it may well be that ours is an era and a culture where the role of pain in human existence is perceived more negatively than ever in recorded history.

I am not suggesting that pain is not negative in the mentioned sense: a force opposing me. What we need to consider as anything but obvious, however, is that the negativity of pain is being judged negatively and only negatively – that whenever something hurts, we are dealing with a type of experience that we should be without, and that we ought therefore to do everything in our power – individually and collectively, employing all means accessible from the domains of culture, science and medicine – to remove it from human existence.

The prevalence of the notion that pain is to be prevented by all means available is revealingly brought out in the World Health Organization's (WHO) definition of health as an optimum human state: "health" means the complete absence of pain and discomfort. The positivity of health is based on the assumed absolute negativity of pain. Therefore, the most ambitious goal for health is attained when pain, its enemy and opposite, is combated until it is eliminated. What the WHO definition of health amounts to, then, is a declaration of war against pain, that is, against its manifestations in so many forms of human suffering. The declaration of war against pain is supported and articulated by modern medicine, refusing to admit "defeat" in the face of suffering – illnesses – which lead to death; the ambition to develop an effective cure against cancer being a case in point. Tellingly, the WHO was headed by a politician originally trained as a physician at the time it launched the definition cited, the former Norwegian prime minister Gro Harlem Brundtland.

This understanding of health illustrates a lot, not only about the WHO but about present-day society. If by "pain" is meant everything that hurts, and if everything that hurts is considered undesirable, it seems logical to concentrate all available resources and knowledge on winning the fight against pain – winning it once and for all, as it were, on behalf of humanity, thereby securing for us a bright future, one where pain no longer spells destiny and doom, or cannot be eliminated. In other words, suffering, as a direct consequence of pain, is in principle generally *preventable*. And since it is so in principle – itself a cultural notion – all good forces are seen as entitled to join in making it so in practice. Indeed, who can reasonably be opposed to advances in medical science, and the technologies it employs and helps revolutionize, in its fight against all kinds of disease, considering pain induced by disease not only as something wholly negative but as something that needs not exist, that one day shall exist no more? Who would turn down the possibility of being helped by advances in medicine if accepting the help they offer means saving (or prolonging) one's life, or that of a loved one? Given this conception, there seems to be no rational grounds on which to oppose a fight against the negativity of pain that holds the promise of success.

Notwithstanding the apparent implausibility of opposing the prevailing wholesale negative view of pain, in the following I shall set out some reasons to question it. This prompts the question of what an alternative view will amount to. Will it be a simple negation, stating that pain is (to some extent and in some respect) good, that it contains something of genuine positive value, without which we would somehow be poorer and worse off?

To start considering a view of pain that refuses to see it as wholly and exclusively negative in human life, we need to ask whether it is true that we only experience pain as, by experience, undesired and principally undesirable, hence wholly and intrinsically negative.

To be sure, if the axe hits my leg, the blow *is* painful, it *does* hurt, and all I want then and there is for the pain to stop, as quickly as possible and whatever it takes. Why want anything that is painful? Indeed, why question what appears as one of the most obvious and irrefutable facts in human existence: that the pain anyone suffers is experienced as unequivocally unwanted, and therefore something to be deemed negative, unanimously and indisputably so?

In my view, to determine the character of pain and to evaluate its significance in human existence on these simple terms would be premature, even mistaken. There is a more fundamental dimension involved that needs to be addressed: As humans we come into the world as *beings exposed to the experience of pain*. Our susceptibility to pain is part of our *conditio humana*, helping define what sort of creatures we are – not only individually, but socially, culturally and – last but not least – morally.

Before examining the implications of this, we need to address the fact that human beings resent and fear pain. To be sure, Jeremy Bentham, the father of utilitarianism – one of the dominant ethical theories of modernity, aptly expressing its mentality – considered it a universal truth that humans will always seek for a maximum reduction of pain and a maximum degree of pleasure: The less the amount of pain encountered in life, the better. The "good" we naturally seek for is a direct offshoot of the desire to lead a life rid of pain, striking it down and minimizing it whenever met upon. The logical ultimate goal, then, is the complete removal of pain as a reality to be endured in human life: The more efficient and sophisticated the means developed to ensure such removal, the better, both individually and for humankind.

Though easily recognizable as a feature of modern life and modern ethics, the Benthamian view is far from covering the whole story. For while it is true that we shun pain, it is equally true that it turns us on, excites us and that we actively seek it – not all the time, to be sure, but at times, thus reminding us that as far as the negatives or positives of pain are concerned, "it depends".

My capacity as a human being to feel pain has multiple functions. On the one end of the spectrum, it alerts me to danger, prompting me to stop, prevent or avoid what might prove fatal to me. To be able to avoid or prevent pain, I need to be capable of perceiving and feeling it, as a possible reality in myself and in others. On the other end, it attracts me like a magnet, prompting me to approach and test the limits of what I can endure without the consequences being fatal – pain as a test case for my character and strength, my tolerance in the face of hardship, my degree of dedication to what I strive for and hope to accomplish, be it for others or purely for myself.

Importantly, this quality of my capacity to feel pain covers both a physical and a psychological (mental and affective) dimension: Whereas experiencing pain as a means of testing my character demonstrates its moral dimension, experiencing it as a means of testing my strength demonstrates its physical one. Indeed, to a considerable extent, showing that one is able to endure a certain amount of pain without collapsing, without giving up the goals one is seeking when encountering pain along the way, is a crucial factor for the assessment of a person's moral character and inner strength. Furthermore, pain also seems to be without any equivalent when it comes to feeling alive: The pain I feel is hard proof, that I am alive and that something is *real*. Pain has a privileged position in our existence in that it shows that what happens to me *matters*: I cannot be indifferent to the presence of pain; its presence – or absence – makes a difference.

This reasoning leads to the following claim: If pain were to be eliminated as a reality (or potentiality) in my life, life would be so much poorer for it. It would be bereft of a crucial criterion of reality, of judging whether something is real and what its reality amounts to, positively or negatively. Principally, the elimination of pain might come about in two ways, outwardly or inwardly, as it were: Either in that pain is removed from external reality (never again shall I be in a situation of encountering pain), or in that my human capacity for experiencing pain (reacting by way of feeling it) is removed so that pain-susceptibility is no longer part of my human repertoire.

On the face of it, both versions of the elimination of pain may seem implausible – lofty notions and speculations rather than real-life options. Even so, it may turn out that this holds merely for the past, and not necessarily for the future. What do I mean by saying so?

To understand what is at issue here, we need to take a closer look at the role of culture in making us, as individuals, assess pain the way we do – doing so being not a matter of (our) nature but always something mediated by culture.

The fact that throughout human history pain has been a crucial feature of the *conditio humana*, ineluctably and inevitably so, means that it has been among the experiential phenomena depicted – in some specific manner – by every known culture. One of the tasks with which any culture has to grapple, on behalf of its members, is to propose a reasonable answer to the existential question: Why is there suffering among humans? To develop a narrative to lend some meaning to the presence of suffering, be it of a religious or secular sort, is part and parcel of the symbolic work performed by a culture, thereby providing each individual member with the means required to articulate how the encounter with pain is experienced, so as to make it something that can be shared with others, enabling them to try to mitigate the pain suffered, be it by medical means or on a purely communicate level, by showing compassion and expressing sympathy. Being, as I observed above, a non-neutral and thus charged phenomenon, pain – that of others as well as my own – calls out for a *common* symbolic framework by which to address and decide upon its meaning, significance and impact in the concrete case, as suffered by a specific person under specific circumstances.

For culture to fulfill this narrative role, the susceptibility to pain of all its human members is taken for granted: Our common humanity is to a large extent based on such susceptibility as a given, equally applicable to all. To recognize this is to appreciate the *moral* significance of pain: Since I am just as susceptible to it as you are, the fact that you are now experiencing it is something I can relate to – it is part of our shared repertoire as human agents and therefore part of what we may meaningfully address and share with each other within a common moral universe. Since pain is no stranger to me, I am no stranger to pain – yours as well as mine. Sharing the condition of exposedness to it means that pain is indispensable in giving each of us access to the reality of the other's weal and woe – access to the moral universe in which we all partake, alternately in the roles of the one in pain and of the other (e.g. patient) from whom a response to pain is required; a response that, depending on the cultural framework both parties share, will be deemed as either appropriate or not, and sanctioned accordingly. Since the very phenomenon of pain is charged, responses to it are as well. Pain does not allow for indifferent or neutral responses and relationships – and that also holds for attempts to denial. To repeat, it is not only that human life as we know it would be poorer absent the reality (actuality and potentiality) of pain; moral life as we practice it would be without a crucial cornerstone as well.

In my view there are five non-optional conditions of human life: dependency, vulnerability, mortality, fragility of (inter-human) relations, and existential loneliness. These are conditions of the way we live our lives in that they (separately or in some combination) pose limits to our quest for autonomy understood as self-sufficiency, as attainment of invulnerability and independence from others. My claim is that by putting a premium on individual autonomy, the culture of present-day society promotes precisely such an ideal of self-sufficiency: of being able, as a fully mature adult, to "master" one's existence without there being any limits to what one can have a successful go at achieving, be it in the form of status or material prosperity, both taken as the rewards to which our efforts ("Leistungen") entitle us.

The cultural primacy granted the demonstrated ability to be an independent, autonomous individual understood as someone who fends for himself, who strives not to be a burden on others, affects the way in which the phenomenon of pain is being perceived. To see how this plays out, we need to distinguish between the kind of pain that is eminently physical – such as the hurt caused by the blow to the leg – and the kind of pain that is either partly or predominantly mental, as in suffering anxiety or depression. Though admittedly too crude to do justice to the fact that pain is often a case of a combination of the two (think of somatization), the distinction marks the difference between pain in the form of injury and pain in the form of offense: As human beings, we can be hurt, and thereupon feel pain, in two major ways – *either* by bodily harm, whereby the cause is a concrete, visible event (the axe blow again, or being hit by another person), *or* by being insulted and humiliated in ways inducing (nonphysical) loss or defeat, something that may assume either a manifest form (the offensive remark you made about me) or an invisible and so purely negative one (being overlooked by others). The mental pain I am getting at is the pain produced by what is experienced as a blow against one's self-worth: namely, by being ignored as someone commanding respect, as someone entitled to being taken seriously as a human agent with distinct intentions, feelings, and ventures in the world; in short, as an inviolable agent according to Kant. Although it surely is painful to be contradicted by others, by their resistance to what I express or hope to achieve; but being overlooked and in that sense "invisible", being nobody to them, may be even worse in terms of the mental pain suffered.

Factoring out for now instances of self-harm, what follows from the fact that humans can be hurt in these two ways – by being physically harmed or by being ignored?

Before answering, we need to observe that the distinction is far from exhaustive: Pain resulting from illness such as cancer is not included. Indeed, much of the suffering that goes with the somatic diseases treated by traditional medicine is left out. By contrast, my chosen focus here is on the kinds of pain that

I typically suffer at the hands of others – whereby the depth of the hurt, the sting if you like, is a direct consequence of someone's deliberate wish to hurt me. Nothing hurts more than the pain inflicted by some other person with the explicit wish to hurt me.

Above I noted that the shared susceptibility to pain is a cornerstone of inter-human morality. Pain is a source of solidarity inasmuch as we are not strangers to each other's pain. However, as we now recognize, the experience-based insight each of us has into what pain amounts to is twofold: Either we may choose to do our best to protect the other against its reality; or we may choose the opposite, to exploit that common susceptibility, that first-person knowledge about what pain feels like, so as to hurt the other where we expect it to hurt the most. Our shared vulnerability-based predicament may prompt immoral acts, including sadism and downright evil, just as it may prompt moral ones, like expressing concern, compassion and respect.

Mental pain of the kind that involves reduced agency, vitality and self-worth as a direct result of inflictions by others can be handled by the individual in two ways: either by seeking to rid oneself of the discomfort suffered by *transporting* it onto others, by causing *them* to suffer according to the logic that the more I cause others to suffer, the less I suffer myself, as if the distribution of pain were a zero-sum-game. To transport pain by way of shifting it from myself onto another person means to treat it as an object, something that can me moved from one place (person) to the other. Causing the other to be in pain holds the promise of gaining mastery, of being in control; unfolding full agency by way of forcing the other to suffer as one's victim – as though enjoying being a fully autonomous subject is possible only at the price of making the other into an object. This may sound farfetched and primitive. Yet frank reflection tells us that it is something we all (sometimes) engage in: To rid myself of the "low" caused by my colleague's sarcastic remark as I was leaving the office, I throw an insult at my wife back home, hoping for relief as a result of shifting the pain away from myself, treating it like garbage.

There is, thank God, an alternative strategy. Instead of seeking to transport the reality of pain from myself onto others, I may engage in its *transformation*. To transform pain means to articulate it symbolically so as to communicate it – not the pain as such, but what it means to me to experience it – to others. This requires trust in the fact that pain is indeed a human experience that *can* be shared with others, that my pain is not unintelligible or inaccessible to them, but something to which they can meaningfully relate. Their doing so ("I understand how you feel, given what happened to you") allows me to experience relief (through communicative sharing) from the sting of the pain, from suffering it in isolation – a relief that is also sought by the alternative strategy of transportation, yet in that case futilely and destructively so, since making others suffer at least as much as I do (did) is as ineffective (in the long run) as it is immature: Far from being a strategy that successfully defeats or overcomes pain, putting an end to it, transportation helps prolong and amplify it by "sending" the burden to others, prompting them in turn to seek for chances to shift it onto others yet, causing cycles of violence, be it between individuals or between groups.

For the more mature strategy of transformation to prevail over transportation, however, we as individuals need the symbolic communication resources provided by our common culture. As mentioned above, cultures present their members with a certain narrative about pain, promoting ways of evaluating it and dealing with it in regard to others, inasmuch as pain is a universal given – hence topic of concern – in human existence: a phenomenon bound to materialize, sooner or later, in every person's life. Triggers for pain in my life may vary from those in yours: In my case it may be, presently, the divorce I am going through; in yours the sudden death of your sister; in our common friend's case, his being dismissed from his job. And so on and so forth. Whereas my divorce illustrates the condition I referred to as "the precariousness of our relations", the death of a sibling illustrates that of mortality as well, reminding me of my own mortality as part of the loss induced; whereas losing one's job illustrates the condition of dependence – being threatened as far as the ability to "keep going", to keep afloat economically (but more generally as well), is concerned. Depending on the nature of the condition actualized, some variant of mental pain will be experienced, leading perhaps to anxiety and depression if allowed to develop according to its own emotional logic, lest it be contained, communicatively, in a manner involving transformation (as opposed to transportation) in the given sense.

> Yes, I was absolutely shattered when it happened; everything looked bleak and I lost faith in myself, in there being a meaningful future for me. But then sharing the pain of the blow I had suffered with a friend, and also reading a novel depicting a character I could easily identify with, besides returning to the music that I always took some comfort in listening to, slowly combined to have an effect on me: I still felt low, but no longer in a way that posed an existential threat. I found that I could go on living despite – even with – what happened.

The importance of the role played by culture turns on how the five conditions I have presented are thematized, normatively as well as descriptively: as the universal givens marking the boundaries within which all individual human lives are lived, boundaries we simply have to observe and respect; or, alternatively, as something wholly negative, posing limits only seemingly definitive and irre-movable, hence something we should seek to avoid and to minimize whenever we encounter them, deeming features revealing our vulnerability as a threat not only against flourishing but against our very quest for meaning.

It is to be regretted that current cultural trends help entrench the second narrative rather than the first. In a highly individualized society such as ours, the effect is that life situations involving pain will be perceived as something the affected individual must cope with alone; something that triggers feelings of shame inasmuch as anything that reduces the ability to come forward as fully autonomous, as fit for fight in a highly competitive "winner-takes-all"-society, is a blow to the person's self-esteem and prospects of gaining the rec-ognition of others. To the extent that pain slows us down, that suffering drains our energy and leaves little or nothing left in terms of vitality to excel in a soci-ety where one's status is measured by one's performance on so many competi-tive fields, the reality of pain in human life has become a much heavier burden than it used to be – and needs to be. What is called for is a renewed apprecia-tion of the way in which our shared vulnerability – far from being a sign of weakness, and as such to be feared and resented – is the source of our common humanity and as such an indispensable yet precarious source of morality.

"... somewhere very close to me ..."

Aspects of an Anthropology of Suffering: The Transformative Passivity of Aesthetic Experience

Knut Wenzel

And I, I don't mind the pain (Dylan)

A God does not suffer. *Apatheia* is a quality attributed to God in the philosophical idiom of the *Stoa*, as is *ataraxia* in that of Epicurean philosophy. *Passion* – would mean to be impressed by an external other, hence convertibility, hence cutback in sovereignty, all summing up to: weakness. A God who shall vouch for the stability of a world experienced as being precarious must not be weak. A passionate God is a weak God is a failed God. As the guarantor of the durability and reliability of a world, which human experience encounters as both, endangered and dangerous, God has to be conceived as unimpressed by the condition of that very world. It is the firm that leaves an impression in the soft, the seal in the wax. The impressed is always indulgent. Indulgence is a mode of passivity.[1]

The word *passion* bears knowledge of the connection of lust and woe, not in terms of identity, but of a continuity spanning across a wide landskip of feeling and meaning. *Passivity* undergoes an opposite dialectics in either pole: Desire, being an originally productive activity, struggles for the experience of fulfilment, that is of utmost passivity; suffering, on the other hand, is never only the objective state of being hurt – of inflicted passivity upon me – but is the subjective and active state of experiencing this violation and relating to it at the same time. As the experience of a violation inflicting passivity, suffering immediately inscribes itself into the relation of humans to themselves, or rather comes into its own within the self-relation of the subject. This relation of the subject to itself should not be thought of as a primordial state of stability, nor can it be reduced to a mere transcendental condition of possibility.

---

1 If this piece was to be a theology of suffering, *theo*logy taken in the strict sense of the word, it would have to include central explorations of the thoughts of Jürgen Moltmann (cf. Moltmann 1993) and especially of Kazoh Kitamori, whose "Theology of the Pain of God" (Kitamori 1965) could take advantage of the Japanese translation of Jer 31:20, which reads "My heart pains" instead of: "My heart yearns", thus producing a notion of God most converse to the metaphysical concept of an apathetic God taken as point of departure above.

© BRILL SCHÖNINGH, 2022 | DOI:10.30965/9783657715428_003

It is, instead, subject to what Michel Foucault conceived of as *le souci de soi*, the anthropological task of self-concern (Foucault 1984). As such, it has to be maintained permanently; the human subject may be regarded as constituted not prior to but within this abiding concern to attain themselves in the first place. It is this basic subject-activity – it can be conceived of as *self-conscious liveliness –*, into which the passivity of suffering inscribes itself. Such considerations towards an understanding of suffering by way of subject-theory receive some confirmation from Viktor von Weizsäcker's medical anthropology, with first attempts dating back to some papers from 1927 (Weizsäcker 1926/27 (1987); Weizsäcker 1927 (2008)) and reaching forth to the last great work from 1957, a *pathosophy* (Weizsäcker 2005); throughout his intellectual lifetime Weizsäcker has dedicated his work to the elaboration of an anthropology of the *pathic human*.

Subjectivity is understood best as *presence of the self*: a state of self-presence that is constituted both in an intense and conscious *alertness* and in a profound *submersion* in the constitutional grounds[2] of one's own existence. Thus constituted, the human self is exposed to any object of attention, to being penetrated instantaneously by it right down into the (non-) grounds of existence. This is not happening to the self: the immediate connection of a radical state of attentiveness and the (non-) grounds of existence that becomes manifest in each act of perception is – the very self. Perception, cognition, experience that conveys external reality at once into the deepest grounds of the perceptive self, engrossing it completely, is – suffering. Insofar as it pierces into the surface of self-identity and punches through down as far as to the constitutional grounds of the self's existence, experience is painful: is suffering. In this general scale, taken as, or in continuity to, experience itself, suffering cannot be seen as pathological from the outset – unless the *condition humaine* as such is regarded as pathological.

Only constrictively anyway, only selectively and temporarily are we able to deliberately manage our capability of perception in such a way that we can control the degree by which reality intrudes upon ourselves. We cannot shut our ears; the sense of taste, the sense of touch – they never stop to sense (unless traumatized); and how long will we be able to keep our eyes shut in face of a light that longs to be seen. And this measures only the sensuous spectre of our constitutional openness towards the world. Can we ever cease from feeling, from having reality, be it of exterior or interior quality, that is present in the

---

2   The notion of *grounds* intended here would rather signify those grounds as abysmal, without foundation, as negativistic grounds like they are conceived of in a tradition from Jakob Böhme to Friedrich Schelling (at least) as *Ungrund* (non-grounds).

inner space of resonance which is our soul? Can we ever cease from cognitively reacting to this presence of reality within us? Concentration is, when successful, the gift of modulating our essential world-openness, but not its domination. On each layer of our physical, psychic, and cognitive perception we are impressible. This is true insofar as our capability of perception is unhurt. If the availment of this capability occupies us down to the fundaments of our existence – so that it can be identified as suffering –, we are *possible*, we are capable to suffer in the state of soundness.

These considerations suggest deducing suffering not from the dysfunctional, be this physical, moral or existential, to recognize suffering not as negation of a per se or otherwise good, productive and satisfying continuum of life, but as a radical realization of it. This opens a scope of interpretation of what counts as ill and what as sound, what as harm and what as well-being, and to think this as pleated into one another rather than as simple opposition. Hans-Georg Gadamer has rejected the plain antithetic determination of illness and health by speaking of the "delitescence of health" ("Verborgenheit der Gesundheit"), of the objective indeterminacy of health. In what obtains validity immediately, in illness, health is covertly present, but cannot be determined by itself (Gadamer 1993, 133-148). Gadamer of course does not go so far as to reassess illness as something eligible; illness remains the reason for taking the line of healing, for people becoming patients and getting into medical treatment, for an overall societal discourse, policy, economy, and industry of health care and medical research. However, if health is clandestine, illness as well suffers the loss of a clear-cut definition. All the more important becomes the statement of the human concerned: the ill, the patient, the suffering. But even this statement can pass through revision with the patient undergoing medical treatment.

To Gadamer, there are no objective parameters for a measurement of health. Strictly speaking, health is not an objective matter of fact, but a subjective one. When it is about to identify health, the subject is the entity to turn to; hence the identification of health will always be at the discretion of the individual. Is illness then, in contrast, an objective fact? Suffering and pain at least, which are to a certain degree associated with illness, but reach beyond it and have particular qualities independent from illness, cannot be valued objectively, without referring to the self. Even to suffer and to regard one's suffering as cureless has to be regarded as a Self's statement to suffering, given namely in Leonard Cohen's Song *There ain't No Cure For Love*.[3] A subject's statement as insight into hopelessness or incurability: How can this be? It can be on that

---

3   Included in the Album I'm Your Man from 1988.

account that this respective Self experiences her- or himself as substantially entangled in suffering and pain in such a way that she or he would perceive a surrender of this "illness" to therapy as turning away from the reason of this suffering and, in consequence, as self-abandonment. Suffering, pain, can be tremendously close, an intimate foreign matter, worn in the heart; to eliminate this would mean to be one's own *arrache-cœur* (Vian 1953) or heart snatcher. *The pain is very, very close to me*, the *Violent Femmes* sing in their Song *Nothing Worth Living For*.[4] A manifestation of despair, and an adjuration of salvation at the same time – *There's nothing worth living for tonight/Tell me that there's something worth living for tonight/Don't let me down/Don't let me drown* – it is impossible to dissociate the pain, it is impossible to localize it: *The pain is somewhere/Somewhere very close to me/The pain is somewhere/Somewhere very close to me* – pain is so close to me, it is a closeness without topology – *somewhere very close to me* – it is closer to me than I am to myself, *interior intimo meo*: the position Augustine reserved for God (cf. Augustine, confessions 3.6.11) is here captured by pain. – How could I have this suffering taken away from me, if it is only me to be right inside this pain?

One can be deeply immersed in pain, surrounded by pain, as if sunken in a delirium, caught in a tight cave or submerged under water.[5] Not even then the feeling – taken as the entirety of perception – implodes under the vehemence of pain or fuses with it. It is this unique situation of being-in-pain that even then can still be perceived: a final difference to pain maintained to the last within this being-in-pain. There is something about us which is not overwhelmed by pain while we are overwhelmed by pain. Possibly, this is the virtual basis of the efficacy of torture: The suffering Self not only is exposed to but specifically feels – bodily recognizes – the suffering. Torture exploits this sublime difference and makes the Self endures their suffering. Being in pain creates particular states of consciousness: extreme commitments, or exposures, which at the same time involve extreme dissolutions; abrogated proportions, attributions made impossible, dizziness, indeterminate, unutterable insights crop

---

4   Included in the album 3 from 1988.

5   Think of the enchanting description of a veritable landscape of illness, Virginia Woolf displays in the beginning of her essay "On being ill": "Considering how common illness is, how tremendous the spiritual change that it brings, how astonishing, when the lights of health go down, the undiscovered countries that are then disclosed, what wastes and deserts of the soul a slight attack of influenza brings to view, what precipices and lawns sprinkled with bright flowers a little rise of temperature reveals, what ancient and obdurate oaks are uprooted in us by the act of sickness, how we go down into the pit of death and feel the waters of annihilation close above our heads and wake thinking to find ourselves in the presence of the angels ..., it becomes strange indeed that illness has not taken its place with love and battle and jealousy among the prime themes of literature." (Woolf 2012, 3f.).

up, twirls of truths, complete synaesthesia; all this seems to be incorporated in the scream of pain Edvard Munch has painted four times (plus one lithography he has drawn) between 1893 and 1910: scream of the pain of life.[6] Later, on the stable ground of sobriety, which an abating, afore all-inflating boost of pain may give free, there might arise names: vision, ecstasy, inspiration, revelation. – Being in pain holds insights that are impossible to justify discursively, they remain erratic; their language would be, if at all, not the notional, reasonable discourse but the poem, possibly.

In a letter to her friend, fellow poet, and first biographer, Anne Stevenson, Elizabeth Bishop expresses a dense version of her poetological credo, or her aesthetic theory. She writes: „What one seems to want in art, in experiencing it, is the same thing that is necessary for its creation, a *self-forgetful, perfectly useless concentration.*" (Bishop 1964 (2008)) This is the precondition for productivity, or creativity, in the arts: to be perfectly concentrated but in a fairly unfeasible manner: without focus, aimlessly. Instead, the Self gets involved in this mode of perception. This turns out to be interrelated; Bishop is very precisely here, not only as a poet, whose job it is to care about the words, but philosophically. In fact, she describes a general, an anthropologically significant mode of perception, and not just a technique of poetical productivity. It is this very mode, or dimension, or "layer" of perception which can be called *aesthetic experience*. So, what Bishop actually does is giving a precise definition of aesthetic experience (in its dispositional dimension): self-forgetful, perfectly useless concentration.

Since in a distinctive theoretical shift, which forms an epoch on its own, as it begins pretty much with Immanuel Kant and moves on to the mid-20th century, the focus of aesthetics, of aesthetic theory, has changed from an aesthetics of the art towards an aesthetics of experience, the notion of aesthetic experience is crucial to aesthetic theory. This fundamental turn of perspective has been accompanied by an uncoupling of "the aesthetics" from the art and by its generalization, namely by an anthropologization, or subjectivation, of the aesthetics. Such development notwithstanding, it is vitally debated how to shape a general definition of aesthetic experience. I am not going to go through all these debates here, there is loads of literature about them. A definition of aesthetic experience depends very much on whether you are an American Pragmatist (John Dewey) or a German Idealist (Dieter Henrich), a scholar of the fine arts or of the performing arts, a Derrida-rist or a neuro-scientist. Surprisingly enough – or rather a profound significance – the point Bishop makes is positioned in close neighbourhood with an aesthetic philosophy

---

6   Munch himself gave it the German title: *Der Schrei der Natur.*

which Frankfurt-based philosopher Christoph Menke has been unfolding during the last twenty years, and still is developing further into new directions. With Derrida as one point of departure, Menke develops a notion of aesthetic experience by working through the history of aesthetic theory of Baumgarten, Herder and Kant, Nietzsche, and all the way up to Adorno.

According to Bishop, aesthetic experience is a reflexive experience; in making an experience of this sort, the subject realizes explicitly a relation to itself. But what is more, both relations constituting an aesthetic experience – the object-related and the subject-reflexive – are determined by a negative moment – the *perfect uselessness* of concentration, the *forgetfulness* that coins the reflexive relation of the subject. This double-moment of negativity is crucial to aesthetic experience. What is negated here? Neither the alertness as a habitus necessary for any emphatic act of perception or experience, nor the self as such. In fact, it is a stance of poised disposition that is negated. In aesthetic experience, concentration rather befalls a person, than it being pursued intentionally by them.

In his late writings, Paul Ricœur has worked out a philosophical anthropology latent in his work from the earliest texts onwards, namely the concept of the human as *homme capable*, as capable human. Here, in the perspective of Elizabeth Bishop, we encounter a subject, whose basically – anthropologically – positive attitude regarding its capability is punctuated by a negative moment. It is the same with the self-presence of the subject *within* this experience. Bishop is, to say it again, very precise at this point: Self-presence in the mode of forgetfulness. This basic, subjective oblivion is also blueprinting the attention: concentrating in such a manner as to be unaware of the act of concentration.

Bishop transforms capability into a dialectics of negativity in order to let its creativity become productive – to experience the art of a poem, as author and reader likewise, one has to be concentrated in this negative modulation. Ricœur for his part correlates in his very first proper publication the will – the acme of capability – with the *involontaire*, the involuntary, without which a philosophy of the will would be deficient (Ricœur 1950 (1966)). Menke holds, arguing on the very same line, that a concept of the human as being capable would be substantially incomplete when only grounded on the actual abilities. What we need, in order to execute our abilities, is a resource of force/energy. In tracing the history of aesthetic theory back to Johann Gottfried Herder and beyond, he comes up with the dialectics of capability and force/energy, of "Vermögen and Kraft", constituting subjectivity (Menke 2012).

The notion of force/energy – Kraft – he takes from Herder. Herder, his conversational personality notwithstanding, is a theorist of the profound dimensions of the soul. This can be witnessed, when, in his "Treatise on the origin of language" (Abhandlung über den Ursprung der Sprache, Herder 1772), he identifies the origin of language as lying neither evolutionary in animal proto-languages nor theologically in a divine linguistic initiative – which have been the options of his time – but, anthropologically, or psychologically, in what he calls the silent self-concept of the soul (das stille Selbst-Verständnis der Seele). Language grounds in something non-, or pre-lingual. – The same can be encountered, when he postulates that language arises out of the – intrinsically wordless – profound movements of the soul, speaking of the "free play of the dark forces/energies of the soul" (das freie Spiel der dunklen Seelenkräfte). Free they are from all intention, purpose, meaning, control. At the same time, they are the indispensable conditions (Ermöglichungsbedingung) of our capabilities with which we execute our intentions, purposes, etc. Herder's idea precedes, of course, the emergence of a psychology and psychoanalysis that match the standards we might judge as scientific. But perhaps we should be cautious of evaluating concepts, ideas, intuitions dating from a prescientific era with an all too narrow paradigm of scientific ratio, accepting only what fits instantaneously into it and discarding the rest.

Herder, anyhow, conceives of the soul – of the human as subject in its core – as being constituted by the two principles of Vermögen (capability) and Kraft (force/energy), interrelated in a dialectic dynamics. Whereas the capability is dependent on force/energy as a resource, force/energy on the other hand is no resource but a dimension in itself. Only due to this undisposability it can be a resource. It is this dialectic dynamics of a capability, dependent on force/energy, which in return stands in no functional relationship to our capabilities, that shows a close analogy to Elisabeth Bishop's self-forgetful, perfectly useless concentration. There is a moment of passivity dialectically connected to or interwoven with the capability to be creative; and there is a dimension of "heteronomy" dialectically connected to or interwoven with the subject-autonomy – to make it work, respectively: passivity – the capability; "heteronomy" – the autonomy.

To use the term "heteronomy" at this point is exaggerative, obviously. What is called heteronomous – Kraft/force/energy – is an element at the constitutive core of subjectivity. So, it cannot be called heteronomous in the strict sense of "prescribing a coercive law from an extrinsic stance". But the subject-constitutive dimension of force/energy is by no means at hand to the respective subject executing their capability. This is, why Bishop rightly – and not only in a trivial metaphorical sense – speaks of self-forgetfulness: The one who wants to open her- or himself towards the well of creativity has to "forget" her- or himself. Self-forgetfulness, then, is a mode of self-realization. To relate to one-self in the mode of forgetfulness means to loosen somehow the grid patterns of self-realization – to be concentrated, but uselessly. According to Bishop, there lies perfection in this self-looseness rather than in total self-possession.

We can experience situations of loosened external and internal control, loosened focus, loosened grip. Such situations are part of our basic anthropologically configuration – and they are universally present in human cultures. Ethnologists like Arnold van Gennep and Victor Turner have identified them in rites of passage. They discern three consecutive stages: the stage of separation in which those undergoing these rites loosen their former status, the stage of transition in which they are disturbingly bare of orientation, the stage of incorporation in which they find a new social and psychological anchorage. Turner fixed "preliminal", "liminal", and "postliminal" as nomenclature of the three stages of the rites of passage, signalizing only by terminology the preponderance of the liminal stage (Turner 1967). Cultural theorists like Erika Fischer-Lichte adapted this ethnographical concept in order to describe aesthetic experience, albeit only in relation to the perception of art: watching a play in theatre, or a movie, watching a dance performance, listening to a symphonic or chamber piece of music, reading a poem (Fischer-Lichte 2003; Achille et al. 2012).

Two decisive alterations have been conducted in this adaption. The liminal stage whose preponderance already foreshadowed in Turners nomenclature, but which still was only the middle part of a triple in the rites of passage, receives, as aesthetic experience, primary, if not exclusive, importance. Furthermore, and going along with this, the liminal stage, taken as aesthetic experience, has undergone a reinterpretation in its quality. No longer is it only the transitory middle part of a horizontal syntagma, an interruption, a threshold. Rather, it is regarded as a reality of its own: the feeling of being overwhelmed by a situation, be it of inner or outer origin, which is loosening, unfastening all systems of self-control and self-possession, which is weakening (but not destroying) my life force, which is nebulizing my ability of orientation, hijacking my words, pulling the rug out from under my self-confidence – which is turning my health upside down. This is ambivalent, no doubt. The liminal stage ranges from religious rites to the experience of art, to plain illness. And it apparently is a truism that illness is something negative.

But there is one continual dimension throughout the whole field: a widening of the inner space of experience – as if a gradual annulment of conversant life-structures not necessarily or not only has a damaging or destructive impact, but instead or also is opening a wider space of experience. The interior resonance of experience receives a spatial shape, not that of a defined space – a room –, but rather that of a void: limitless space. This might be the experiential – or phenomenological – fundament of the metaphysical and mystical idea to mirror the cosmos – as the outer space in its entirety – in the human soul as a cosmos interior to the human subject. However, it is significant for the whole complex of aesthetic experience that precisely on the crossroads of religion, mysticism, and modern art there has been developed a theory of experience working with the same spatial shaping: Georges Bataille's *L'expérience intérieure*. Bataille writes: "I call experience a journey to the end of human possibilities. Everyone is free to not undertake this journey. But when he or she does, this means that the existing authorities and values which restrict the possible, are to be neglected."[7] (Bataille 1953 (2017), 14).

This journey we undertake in a liminal stage, or in an aesthetic experience, is all but following a route with its definite start and finish. It is a kind of floating. In a recent study on Beckett and Hölderlin, Dieter Henrich refers to records both from Hölderlin and Rousseau, who remember the identical experience of lying in a boat, watching only the cloudless sky (or should I, in reference to John Lennon say: heaven?), while floating slowly on a lake – and sample this as experience of superabundance. Henrich interrelates this with Beckett's comment on Hölderlin's record, saying that beyond this experience of floating there is only – nothingness. According to Henrich, this does not mean that Beckett has misunderstood Hölderlin, but that his notion of nothingness and Hölderlin's notion of Being fall into one (Henrich 2016).

Whatever is to be said about the metaphysical implications of this – not only is here a noteworthy impregnation of an experience of plenitude with a high degree of passivity to be noticed; moreover delivers the narrated scene an illuminative image of aesthetic experience as an experience of lost orientation, or a stage in which there is no need of orientation, at least for some time. Fischer-Lichte interprets the liminal stage as "Zwischenzustand", as being betwixt everything, which inversely means: not belonging to anything. The liminality is the very topos, on which aesthetic experience is possible, a non-topos: utopia, or a metonymically ever-shifting topos: a hetero-topos (Michel Foucault). Whatever will be experienced in this stage, will be of new shape, uncommon, uncanny even, unsettling like the experience of a young woman or man passing through some rite of passage. Exciting unexpectedness of what is to come, in combination with a condition of passivity – is what makes an aesthetic experience.

A clean separation of the sane and the other is impossible in this field. The aesthetic experience subverts any purpose-focused rationality. From a rational point of view, such a state of mind, or, better said, stage of feeling might seem

---

7 My translation from the German translation.

unsound anyway. – The unsound ground, reversely, may hold the potential of a new beginning, a new reading, of the unpredictable, coming out of nowhere.

Finally, it might sound unsound to say that also in illness, even pain, there is a dimension of aesthetic experience. Scholars as different from each other as Victor von Weizsäcker and Ludwig Wittgenstein argue that it is better – healthier, so to say – not to dissociate illness from the configuration of our Self we can identify with, but to accept it as a meaningful mode of self-realization. Weizsäcker, founder of psychosomatic medicine and author of a medical anthropology, not immediately reaches out for remedy and therapy but asks: What is the determination of this respective disease? I am not going to follow this path. Still, it indicates that there is space for more perspectives on illness apart from a purely negative and technical-therapeutic one. Illness weakens my life force, it drowns my discursiveness in a sea of silence, it veils my mind with colours, sounds, images I didn't want to realize before, and by that, illness prepares the very conditions for or of aesthetic experience. Even pain, severe pain, can amidst its ferocity shift into a thin line of unbound feeling. In illness we are ill, and pain aches, there is no doubt about that. But being in such states of negativity, we are not in principle completely extradited to this. Even under the vehemence of illness and pain we can, maybe even more distinctively than in conditions of health, experience ourselves – albeit in a stage of profound passivity: an experience, the content of which is determined nearly void: we are, life is, in illness, in pain.

This might, it was said, be subject rather of a poem than of a notional discourse – of a poem like the one at the beginning of John Henry Newman's great last poetic work, *The Dream Of Gerontius* from 1865 (Newman 2012); the awareness of death come close is not carried back to the accompanying perceptions of physical misery but stretches out to a feeling absolutely new, yet so, that it all is interleaved by invocations of Jesus and Maria for succour; in their entirety, these lines occur as a single articulation of absolute insecurity:

> Jesu, Maria – I am near to death,
> And Thou art calling me; I know it now.
> Not by the take of this faltering breath,
> This chill at heart, this dampness on my brow, –
> (Jesus, have mercy! Mary, pray for me!)
> 'Tis this new feeling, never felt before,
> (Be with me, Lord, in my extremity!)
> That I am going, that I am no more.
> 'Tis this strange innermost abandonment,
> (Lover of souls! Great God! I look to Thee,)
> This emptying out of each constituent
> And natural force, by which I come to be. (Newman 2012, 6)

For all the singularity, and therefore speechlessness, of an extreme experience of suffering in its inner quality, this respective experience shows structural features, because of which it reads as if seen from the outside. The structure allows to speak of a double outcome of the experience of pain, or suffering.

One such structural feature has already been encountered in that suffering human beings can come across a point from which they virtually, even amidst their being overwhelmed by pain, can turn to this pain.[8] As if within totality – on principle, and in this case within that of the negativity of suffering – there existed a moment of undisposability. As this moment of undisposability within the totality of suffering is an inner reality, its perception can be considered as a true experience of the Self, that is to say, in experiencing undisposability the Self as such becomes subject of their own experience. Even under the smothering load of suffering the Self can find access to traces or veils of a state of non-identity with pain and suffering, allowing to find a relation to suffering instead of being completely lost in it. Insofar as this undisposability is also a quality of the Self's relation to itself, it does not empower the suffering Self to a sovereign position of capability to act in the light of suffering. Subjectivity is not a tool to gain unrestricted self-control. The "activity" opened to the Self by the moment of undisposability – which now can be identified as subject-activity – consists of the ability of not letting yourself be swallowed up completely by the negativity of suffering; it is not more than a last crack, by which a light of the possibility of the other, of other possibilities, might shine into the suffering: a mustard seed of *capabilité* within a cosmos of negativity. And finally: this is all about incarnated subjectivity; its undisposability, its absoluteness, is liable to the limits of an animated finitude. It is precisely physical pain that realizes this liveliness in its vulnerability with an undeniable sharpness, thus laying bare the inner nexus between liveliness and vulnerability. A being is living insofar as it can be hurt, it can die. Suffering demonstrates the value, if not dignity, of a painful, corporeal liveliness by a negativistic, physical persuasiveness.[9]

---

8   Disarmingly simple this is pointed out by Leonard Wayne Sumner: "[H]ow physical pain feels to us, how much it hurts, is one thing; how much it matters to us is another." (Sumner 1999, 106)

9   Cf. Kleinschmidt 2016, 19 with reference to Weizsäcker. That pain presupposes body is central to Lisa Tambornino's philosophy of pain (Tambornino 2013): Tambornino holds "dass sich Schmerzen grundsätzlich dadurch auszeichnen, dass sie im Körper empfunden werden und somit *Introzeptionen* sind" (ibid., 28). Even when Tambornino writes that not the hurt body feels pain but the being the body of which is hurt (ibid., 76), she operates in the framework of a reductionist naturalism; the linkage of the physicalness of pain with the denial of the notion of psychic pain – simply because there is no such a reality as the soul (cf. ibid., 7) – appears, especially in the light of the dynamic developments of the body-mind-debates, as unnecessarily rash.

There is a theological horizon to this moment of undisposability. It can be encountered at a rather prominent locus theologicus: The guilt of Job, what does it consist of? There is no guilt responsible for Job's heavy fate; in this regard, he receives justification against his friends by God. Job's suffering, however, is unjustifiable. Job's actual guilt, as it is disputed between him and God in the last chapters of the book of Job, is that in his complaint against God he totalizes the harm he was exposed to, that he leaves the last word to suffering, that he does not concede any more space to the possibility of a light unhoped for, shedding from elsewhere into the darkness of his misfortune – against all odds. God teaches Job that only one who at least in secret still hopes for an unlikely success, for an unhoped-for rescue can truly be in despair. This is a calculation without learnable method, a calculation of grace that foils all reckoning. God teaches Job that he, who relinquishes the possibility of salvation, relinquishes one's own subjectivity in its undisposability – which is to say: One who relinquishes God as the real possibility of an unexpected meaning that cannot be transferred into a word, a logos, of which the human would be capable of, gives up on himself.[10] This interpretation of suffering finds a New Testament-resonance in the first epistle of Peter. There, the *capabilité* to endure unjustified suffering is named grace: "For this is grace, when, mindful of God, one endures sorrows while suffering unjustly" (1 Peter 2, 19). This does not mean to explain away suffering, but rather to assure that humans have reasons, even if hardly justifiable, to confide and to hope and not to surrender to a view of the world as a completely absurd and meaningless place. Following 1 Peter, grace is to have the strength to hold on to God despite the suffering one experiences. Neither in terms of apportioning of blame nor of theodicy guilt is explained away here. Rather, it is said that amidst a suffering inexplicable and ineluctable (for the time being at least) there is reason to withstand, a reason not to be caught up in suffering. To hold on to this reason, however absurd, is grace of God.[11] – This is one outcome of the experience of suffering.

The other outcome becomes accessible, in a surprising dialectics, via the issue of guilt. It was the inner development of sapiential thought up to Job as a culminating point to resolve the linkage of suffering to guilt. The more astonishing it is to see this linkage return in modern literary-philosophical thought. In his essay "On Pain" from 1934, Ernst Jünger develops a proper metaphysics of pain (Jünger 2008): In a cosmic scale, or at least in one embracing the whole history of humanity, there is an adjustment of well-being and pain at work in

---

10   This roughly paraphrases Paul Ricœur's exegesis of the book of Job given in: Ricœur 1977.
11   Norbert Brox discovers a complete "logic of grace" in 1 Peter. Cf. Brox 1989, 133. In this context Brox quotes Thompson 1966: "Every aspect of life is related to suffering" (ibid., 140).

such a manner that real pain always is the acquittance of a bill of guilt committed elsewhere (Kleinschmidt 2016, 16). Jünger's essay, written in a lucid style and being opaque nonetheless, at least for present day readers, belongs to the work context of the 1932 written comprehensive essay "The Worker" (Jünger 2017), that shows Jünger completing his occupation with extreme right wing ideas, militaristic, anti-democratic, elitist. This occupation he initially exercised politically, shifting to the theoretical-metaphysical edge in the end. "The Worker", and "On Pain" in its wake, unfold a theory of the "new human" which is in fact no more human at all, but a being of the masses, conceived of in analogy to the machines which determine their Lebenswelt: pure will, but with the sensitivity and consciousness having been burnt out, leaving only perfect tractability. The figure of the "worker" could also be described as "soldier". "On Pain" is ostensibly opaque for the polar frostiness with which the totalitarian metaphysics of a post-humanistic world of workers, or soldiers, is displayed. It is profoundly opaque since pain remains astonishingly under-thematized, regarding the text's foreground. Rather, the notion of pain works as a second order-topic in the background of the essay. This architecture – or architexture – reveals Jünger's considerations to be a metaphysics of pain.

The conception of the worker revolves around the vision of a new typos of existence which emerges along with a new level of technical progress, and which supersedes the outworn typos of modernity. A binary anthropology is established; the poles of which differ in their attitude to pain: one is "heroic" (new), the other (old, or "modern"), is characterized by "sensitiveness" (Empfindsamkeit). The sensitive moderns avoid pain by all means, they close their lives away from pain and maintain a non-relation to pain, thus submitting themselves to pain. The "heroic" attitude, by contrast, strives to stay in permanent touch with pain. One who is always primed to confront himself with pain, is free. Discipline, consequently, is defined as "the form by which the human keeps up contact with pain". It is, despite its contamination with right-wing ideology, a cogent critique of modernity, confronting it with its repression and oblivion of pain and suffering, and debunking a societal performance of sensitiveness as the very opposite of a true awareness of suffering and pain. But "keeping up contact with pain" is not necessarily a heroic attitude; it simply is an ambitious stance of humaneness.

Jünger's considerations are remarkable after all in that he places pain in relation to reality in its totality. This is exactly what Victor von Weizsäcker undertakes, also using the notion of guilt, but differently. Weizsäcker's metaphysics of "guilt" operates with the paradigm of anxiety rather than with a heroic one: In the sensation of pain soar night-thoughts; queries and doubts come forward, untampered and wordless, encompassing one's existence as a whole, placing it in an absolute horizon. Thus becomes dubious one's very existence, dubious becomes the horizon itself. Pain turns out to be an experience of difference: as if we eternally owed to "the being" our finitude. This understanding of guilt shows pain as the dark side of our openness towards the whole (Jünger 2017, 18-22). It is the same constellation in which John Henry Newman, in the first lines of Gerontius quoted above, shapes the experience of death come close with the notion of extremity; in the extreme, in the absolute openness of the finite to the whole – without certitude whether it is to the being or to the nothing – there only remains for Gerontius to pray for help.

There is, therefore, a pain, a suffering of our bare being: pain as the irrefutable perception of the tension between finitude and infinity – and as expression of this; our existence necessarily coming with pain – inevitably, incurably.[12]

These remarks might find some confirmation in reflections of Martin Heidegger. Heidegger, who drilled his thoughts ever deeper into the material of thinking by way of reading poems, not only those of Hölderlin, did, on his way into the thick of it, ruminate about pain: not only on the occasion of taking in Georg Trakl's iconic line "Schmerz versteinerte die Schwelle" ("Pain has turned the threshold to stone")[13]; his thinking of pain may have gained an even higher density in reading Stefan George's poem *Das Wort* (*The Word*), written in 1919, included in the highly influential collection *Das Neue Reich* (*The New Realm*) of 1928. I am not going to reconstruct Heidegger's reading of the poem, but only elaborate briefly on the gist of his thinking on pain.[14]

Heidegger's approach is that of philosophical anthropology. The poet struggling with the word represents the human as such. As fundamental moods of the human mind Heidegger identifies joy and grief. Out of the depths of joy wells grief, joy out of an abysmal grief. Pain is the *nomos* of their interplay. Pain tunes the mortal's mind in on the tone of gloom, of a heavy heart. This heart may have a sense of the abundant real – joy – but can never actually have it – grief. The abundant real is close, but in a mode of longing (joy); it is remote in a mode of not having it (grief). And this densely pleated oneness of presence and absence of the abundant real is so acute that it is pain.

In the mood of grief, and of joy, we experience the radical incompleteness of our existence to a physical extend; hence it is in pain we are most intimate with ourselves. Pain is the sentience, as is gloom the mood, of the finitude of

---

12   Significantly Weizsäcker understands the "guilt" he sees given in the experience of pain, in analogy with melancholy; cf. Jünger 2017, 21.

13   The second line in the third verse of the Poem *Ein Winterabend*, 1915.

14   For the following cf. Heidegger 1985, 222f.

our Selves, a finitude of physical, of painful desire; existential pain discloses this finitude as openness of a boundless desire. Following George, Heidegger names this finitude open to infinity, but in the mode of painful desire, *surrender* ("Verzicht"). In surrender we renounce what we commit ourselves to. To be deeply devout to what is absolutely out of reach – is pain: call it religion, or piety.[15] The state of pain, understood in an existential scope, can be called a religious mood insofar as it is affirmed, adopted pain; religion, considered as taking up the perspective of pain, constitutes a negativistic consciousness, a consciousness of the non-identical.

"Kein Ding sei, wo das Wort gebricht" – ("Where word breaks off nothing may be"[16]): Heidegger correctly reads George's poem as poetical rumination about the poet's business and the poet's experience as allegorical representation of the human condition. There is no "thing", no graspable reality without "the word" naming, exposing, identifying reality. In confronting the real the poet, however, lacks the word. This failure turns out to have a positive opening: The lacking of the word, the incapability to grasp reality, to have a grip on it, by means of the word, the negation of having access to the real by disposing of it – the poetic articulation of this impotence is, as such, the utmost affirmation of the real. Affirming the real by not grasping it: It is this aesthetics of uncontrollability (Unverfügbarkeit) that Heidegger excavates out of the experience of pain, a negative dialectics of surrender and longing, which I call the religion of the non-identical. For what else could a recognition that is acted out as surrender be, but an experience in pain, a melancholic mood? Melancholy is hope given up: Hope with no expectations. Terry Eagleton prepends his Page-Barbour-Lectures from 2014 with a quotation from the English Dominican theologian Herbert McCabe as a motto: "We are not optimists; we do not present a lovely vision of the world which everyone is expected to fall in love with. We simply have, wherever we are, some small local task to do, on the side of justice, for the poor." (Eagleton 2015, vii) For McCabe, "we" are the Christians; hope with no expectations is clearly qualified as an attitude of religious faith here, of spiritual poise.

---

15   Religion is the term more common than piety. When I use a word of the semantic field of "religion" here I think of the personal experience rather than of the societal institution and would favour "religion" to sound as "piety", or "faith".

16   From: Gatherings: The Heidegger Circle Annual, 1 (2011): 54-73, 62 (Tranlation: Jussi Backman).

Bibliography

Achille, Jochen/Borgards, Roland/Burrichter, Brigitte (2012): Liminale Anthropologien. Zwischenzeiten, Schwellenphänomene, Zwischenräume in Literatur und Philosophie, Würzburg: Königshausen und Neumann.

Bataille, Georges (2017): Die innere Erfahrung (L'expérience intérieure, 1953), vol. 2, Berlin: Matthes & Seitz.

Bishop, Elizabeth (2008): Letter to Anne Stevenson, January 8th, 1964, in: E. Bishop/R. Giroux (Ed.), Poems, prose, and letters. New York: Library of America, 855-864.

Brox, Norbert (1989): Der erste Petrusbrief, 3rd ed., EKK XXI, Zürich/Neukirchen-Vluyn: Benziger/Neukirchener, 133.

Eagleton, Terry (2015): Hope without Optimism, New Haven-London: Yale University Press.

Fischer-Lichte, Erika (2003): Ästhetische Erfahrung als Schwellenerfahrung, in: J. Küpper/Chr. Menke (Eds.), Dimensionen ästhetischer Erfahrung. Frankfurt: Suhrkamp, 138-161.

Foucault, Michel (1984): Histoire de la sexualité III. Le souci de soi, Paris: Gallimard.

Gadamer, Hans-Georg (1993): Über die Verborgenheit der Gesundheit, Frankfurt: Suhrkamp.

Heidegger, Martin (1985): Das Wort, in: idem, Unterwegs zur Sprache. Gesamtausgabe, vol. 12, Frankfurt: Vittorio Klostermann, 205-225.

Henrich, Dieter (2016): Sein oder Nichts. Erkundungen um Samuel Beckett und Hölderlin, München: Beck.

Herder, Johann Gottfried (1722): Abhandlung über den Ursprung der Sprache, Berlin.

Jünger, Ernst (2008): On pain. Translated and introduced by David C. Durst. With a preface by Russell A. Berman, New York: Telos Press.

Jünger, Ernst (2017): The worker. Dominion and form. Edited by Laurence Paul Hemming. Translated by Bogdan Costea and Laurence Paul Hemming, Evanston (Ill.): Northwestern University Press.

Kitamori, Kazoh (1965): Theology of the pain of God, Richmond/Va.: John Knox Press.

Kleinschmidt, Sebastian (2016): Schmerz als Erlebnis und Erfahrung. Deutungen bei Ernst Jünger und Viktor von Weizsäcker, Warmbronn: Verlag Ulrich Keicher.

Menke, Christoph (2012): Force. A fundamental concept of aesthetic anthropology, New York: Fordham University Press.

Moltmann, Jürgen (1993): The passion of Christ and the suffering of God, in: The Asbury Theological Journal 48, 19-28.

Newman, John Henry (2012): Der Traum des Gerontius. Englisch/Deutsch. Translated by Paul Pattloch, Einsiedeln/Freiburg: Johannes.

Ricœur, Paul (1950): Philosophie de la volonté, T. 1: La volontaire et l'involontaire, Paris: Seuil.

Ricœur, Paul (1966): Freedom and Nature. The Voluntary and the Involuntary. Edited by John Wild et al., Chicago: Northwestern University Press.

Ricœur, Paul (1977): Toward a hermeneutic of the idea of revelation, in: The Harvard Theological Review 70, 1-37.

Sumner, Leonard Wayne (1999): Welfare, happiness and ethics, Oxford: OUP.

Tambornino, Lisa (2013): Schmerz. Über die Beziehung physischer und mentaler Zustände, Berlin-Boston: de Gruyter.

Thompson, J.W. (1966): "Be submissive to your masters": A study of 1 Peter 2:18-25, in: RestQ 9, 66-78.

Turner, Victor W. (1967): Betwixed and between: The liminal period in Rites de Passages, in: The forest of symbols, New York: Cornell University Press.

Vian, Boris (1953): L'arrache-cœur, Paris: Vrille.

Weizsäcker, Viktor von (1987): Der Arzt und der Kranke. Stücke einer medizinischen Anthropologie, in: Viktor von Weizsäcker, Gesammelte Schriften, vol. 5. Edited by P. Achilles. Frankfurt: Suhrkamp.

Weizsäcker, Viktor von (2005): Pathosophie, in: Viktor von Weizsäcker, Gesammelte Schriften, vol. 10. Frankfurt: Suhrkamp.

Weizsäcker, Viktor von (2008): Über medizinische Anthropologie (1927), in: Viktor von Weizsäcker, Warum wird man krank? Ein Lesebuch. Edited by W. Rimpau. Frankfurt: Suhrkamp, 140-163.

Woolf, Virginia (2012): On being ill (1930), Ashfield (Ma.): Paris Press.

The Concept of Suffering in the Context of Palliative Medicine

Bernd Oliver Maier

Palliative Care is a medical approach aimed at the improvement of quality of life and the relief of distressing symptoms associated with life-threatening illnesses. It incorporates a generalist and a specialist perspective. The concept of palliative care should be integrated in a treatment plan for people at end of life. If a complex situation requires complex interventions, access to specialist palliative care should be guaranteed. There are many different guidelines on how this care should be provided, available on a national and international level like "S3 Leitlinie für Menschen mit einer unheilbaren Krebserkrankung" of the German Association for Palliative Care (DGP 2015) or the EAPC (European Association of Palliative Care) framework papers on the use of palliative sedation (Cherny et al. 2009).

The main target of palliative care intervention is the reduction of symptom burden, for the patients. Symptoms in palliative care are generally understood as unpleasant sensations or experiences. They are roughly categorized in four domains: somatic or physical problems, psychosocial problems or spiritual problems. The symptom most frequently associated with symptom burden is pain. Despite a wide range of underlying causes for the experience of pain, it is generally expected to occur more often when approaching death. Therefore, special attention is focused on fighting pain. Often, the word "pain" is used as a verbal expression for a sum of unpleasant experiences associated with dying, touching on underlying causes far beyond pathophysiological patterns. In this context the concept of total pain includes a simultaneous presence of a wide range of contributing factors with somatic, psychological, social and spiritual aspects; in fact it can derive from any individual domain being addressed as relevant to palliative care. The word suffering is synonym with symptom burden. In the official WHO definition, relief of suffering is quoted as a core attitude of palliative care: an "approach that improves the quality of life [...] and the relief of suffering" (WHO). But there is no further explanation about how suffering is defined, diagnosed or treated.

© BRILL SCHÖNINGH, 2022 | DOI:10.30965/9783657715428_004

Meanings of the Word Suffering

Despite widespread use of the word "suffering" in the medical context, suffering is not clearly defined at all in this context. This leaves room for interpretation in all medical fields, but especially in palliative care. Aside from the medical use, suffering is used in a non-medical philosophical context as well as in everyday language. Popular views understand suffering as logical consequence of humans' capacity to cognitively reflect on individual experiences and put them in context of individually graded levels of pleasure. Happiness and pleasure are natural opposites of suffering on an emotional scale. Experiencing happiness is not possible without an idea of how it feels to be unhappy. In contrast, the experience of suffering, as a baseline human experience, is a prerequisite for gaining an idea of how life in its less burdensome times might feel, as a baseline for improvement.

In this context, we are talking about suffering as a non-medical concept; to be heartbroken surely makes people suffer, but is not an accepted medical condition urging medical care. Life events in this sense consistently have the capacity to increase the intensity of suffering, without any underlying medical condition as a trigger. Suffering in this context describes a negative but existential and fundamental emotional experience associated with being human and life in general. Suffering here is fundamental, and possibly even constituting part of human nature. Having accepted this, the question remains, what turns suffering – a possibly normal state of human emotions – into a state urging medical care at the end of life. Also: how the medical concept and the non-medical concept of existential suffering can be applied in a well-balanced therapeutic approach aiming for comfort as a therapeutic goal. This is one of the main challenges of the palliative care approach.

Prerequisites of Palliative Care

Palliative Care, as any medical intervention, is bound to the overall rules of medical procedures. Simplified, in a didactic two-step model, any medical action needs to be grounded on two basic requirements; there has to be a justifying indication in the first step. Second, it requires the informed consent of the patient. Indication is based on a medical professional's judgment, that application of a medical procedure will make a beneficial and meaningful contribution in achieving a relevant goal according to the patient's own perception. To establish an indication, the judgment has to be based on transparent criteria, which are usually the result of diagnostic procedures. This is true for palliative care as for any other medical specialty. In contrast, informed consent does not need any objective criteria. Everyone has a right, and possibly even the obligation, to decide on proposed treatments. This is an act of autonomy. Patients' rights have to be respected. Denial of informed consent for a proposed treatment has to be accepted even if it may appear to be a very unreasonable decision. Consented prerequisites for access to palliative care are: the existence of a diagnosis of a life threatening disease with a limited prognosis, unmet needs in any of the relevant dimensions, and an overall acceptance that medical intervention should aim at least more for quality of life than for length of survival of the patient.

When Does "The End of Life" Begin?

Limited prognosis is thereby regarded as a marker for being near the end of life. But here again we cannot rely on a good definition. What defines being at the end of life? Determinants considered to be relevant are, for example, biological features: diseaserelated expectations of progression towards dying. Pathological findings allow differentiating between various risk groups for disease progression. Last, but not least, the simple fact of age is an important prognostic parameter. The availability of treatment options modifies the impact of the estimated natural course of a disease and therefore is an independent important factor. But what happens if a broadened focus is applied to answer the question? Social factors like a lack of social attachment, impairment of cognitive functions, individual values or religious or spiritual beliefs heavily influence the idea of when "end of life" begins. Whose perception is actually the important one? The one of the affected person, the one of the patient, or the one of the healthcare professional?

Regarding the applicability of potentially lifesaving treatments patient's personal attitudes and beliefs become highly decisive: Motivation for therapy or not consenting to treatment proposals does definitely determine whether someone is near the "end of life". Therefore even in medical decision making the level of personal views and characteristics enters the scene inevitably and is a major influence.

Definitions as Key to Interventions?

In summary, the described lack of consistency in definitions urges an interpretation on an individual basis. The medical framework does not allow for painting the complete picture. For example, concepts of dignity, hope, and comfort challenge medical selfunderstanding, as they are considered to be an integral part of any human interaction and not just medical interventions. General applicability is based in our societies' perception of good lifestyle and does not necessarily need an indication. It implies a moral concept instead of a medical indication. But if the concept of dignity is transformed in a therapeutic concept like, Chochinov's Dignity Therapy (Chochinov 2012), it becomes regulated by the medical framework. Then, an indication is required as justification for delivery of dignity, hope or comfort – and to make sure that reimbursement is made available. Humans approaching death are at risk of being deprived of the normal values of our culture and society. They are perceived as being at risk, especially by being drawn into the treadmill of standardized medical procedures, which often tends to neglect or diminish hope, dignity and comfort. Therefore, as counterpart, medical attention is increasingly drawn on these issues in the form of the palliative care approach, while at the same time the medical system is considered to be the violator. Conflicting and potentially contradictory medical ideas and strategies are within the accepted range of individual approaches in a democratic society. However, a life threatening diagnosis leads to a longing for stability and clarity. The overall amount of information available challenges and destabilizes individuals in a time of open access to information overkill. Information is free, but guidance and orientation is not! Palliative care aims at protecting individuals' values in this time of threat and crisis. It transforms the overall present topic "suffering" into a conceptual medical subject with all implications, chances and risks for misunderstanding.

Can We Measure Suffering?

At the beginning of any medical treatment plan, there has to be a diagnosis based on the clinical presentation and other findings leading to a hypothesis about how the treatment could be tailored most effectively. In the context of palliative care, the focus is less on objective findings like laboratory results of blood samples and images like computer tomographic scans. Focus is shifted to the subjective experience of the patient. Subjective wellbeing outweighs objective findings as a promoter for interventions considered helpful. Therefore, profound exploration of the patient's personal views is a baseline for any intervention targeted at the alleviation of suffering. Socalled "Patient Reported Outcome Measures" (PROMs) are used to assess intensity, character and individually experienced relevance of symptoms in a valid and

standardized way (Bausewein et al. 2016, 6-22). This approach enables professionals to compare different patients as well as individual responses to treatment of a single patient in a timely manner. Established and validated tools
like European Organization for Research and Treatment of Cancer Quality
of Life Questionnaire with Thirty Items (EORTC QLQ 30 Pal), Minimales
Dokumentationssystem (MIDOS), Edmonton Symptom Assessment Scales
(ESAS) and Palliative Outcome Score (POS) touch on suffering by asking
for the presence and severity of certain symptom domains. The majority of
these tools focus on somatic topics. A minority test psychosocial or spiritual
domains. In regular clinical use, the somatic tools are mainly used, the others
are often only applied in a research setting. Coming back to suffering remaining a phenomena not clearly medically defined, it becomes obvious that none
of the tools is especially designed to evaluate the complete complexity of suffering. However, these tools contribute important information as they heighten
the teams' awareness of issues which are not quantifiable and otherwise only
a matter of individual interpretation. Knowledge about strengths and limitations of these assessment tools therefore helps the clinicians to establish an
open and transparent communication with patients, and, furthermore, within
the professional team. Finding a commonly understood language on individual
suffering is one of the most important requirements for effective treatment.

Hierarchy of Needs as a Model for the Change in Medical Perspective

To understand the difficulty of assessing suffering, it might be helpful to put the
usual medical approaches into perspective with suffering. I use the hierarchy
of needs model by Abraham Maslow as a didactic model to illustrate the difficulty in establishing a clear-cut threshold for medical interventions. Maslow
originally invented the hierarchy of needs model for tailoring advertisements.

In the pyramid of needs model, Maslow distinguishes between deficit-
orientated needs and growth-orientated needs. Deficit-orientated needs are
characterized as being baseline needs concerning physiological function and
safety issues. Growth-orientated needs touch on higher cognitive and emotional functions like longing for love and belonging to others, sustaining esteem
and reaching self-actualization. Growth-orientated needs promote the idea of
leading a meaningful and fulfilled life. Using this model in a medical context
of a seriously ill patient, I translate deficit-orientated physiological needs as
somatic symptoms like somatic pain, breathlessness, nausea and others –
which all are unpleasant and should be avoided. Relevant safety issues are, for

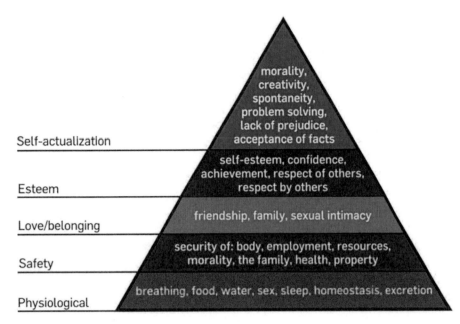

Fig. 3.1   Maslow's Hierarchy of Needs

example, the aim of sustaining a certain standard of living despite not being able to work anymore. Growth-orientated needs remain less directly altered by a diagnosis. Nevertheless they are all put at a high risk of becoming unreachable due to a life threatening disease and its consequences. All deficits in all components together make people suffer. We generally agree on health being more than the absence of illness, even though we do not describe in detail what is meant by that. It relates to an idea of not only avoiding harmful and unpleasant experiences, but aiming for higher goals being naturally implied in human nature. Humans want to be loved, they want to live a meaningful life. We do not generally agree on to what extent it is obligatory to medically address these issues in terms of treatment and supply of resources. It is well acknowledged that avoidance of pain and comparable physiological symptoms is considered a real and important medical task. The medical system addresses social issues like social security as well. But the more issues of the growth-orientated needs' side are addressed, the less they are originally considered to be targets for medical intervention. Palliative Care here is distinguishably different from other medical specialities. The palliative care approach incorporates care for the whole variety of needs, including the growth-orientated perspective. The holistic approach does not allow any upfront priorities. It urges exploration of the patient's perspective and therefore addresses the well accepted medical

side of suffering and the less medicalized existential side of suffering at the
same time.

Dimensions of Suffering

The dimensions of suffering can be categorized according to their profile of
general acceptance within the medical field.

a)   *Socio-biological Symptoms*

Symptomatic burden due to pathological somatic conditions, like dsypnea
due to pleural effusions or a low hemoglobin level, is attributed as being medically relevant and urging imminent medical action or intervention for relief
of suffering. Equally – even if contentwise already linked closer to existential issues – symptomatic burden due to classified psychiatric disorders, like
manifest major depression, is regarded as another area of imminent medical
concern. There is an idea and understanding that symptomatic burden due to
lack of social resources is an area of interest, though, for example, in Germany
exhaustion of social support systems is not accepted as a reason for hospital
admission. It is regarded as an issue for support services, but not in the core
focus of medical attention.

b)   *Existential Symptoms*

Symptomatic burden due to existential distress, like not feeling of any value
often is not regarded as a symptom requiring special support, but is often considered to be a logical consequence (and, therefore, almost normal) in the context of life-threatening disease or end of life care (like pain was regarded as
obligatory phenomena and not a treatable symptom when dying only some
decades ago). This classification reveals an important difference in the pure
likelihood of medical reaction to suffering in association with the underlying
causes.

Real Life Relevance of the Difference of Socio-biological and
Existential Symptoms

In real life, the situation is more complex. Most commonly, there are multiple
symptoms present at the same time, and the underlying causes are not easily
identified. Even if they are hypothetically identified, the relevance of the different contributing factors might be judged differently by the patient and the

health care professionals. Again, only effective communication can bridge this gap and avoid ending up in pitfalls such as paternalistic approaches. Looking at resources, the differentiation illustrates that aside of the well-accepted area of medical attention, the somatic side of suffering, no reliable concept of adequate medical support for existential distress exists. In conclusion, suffering in palliative care can be conceptualized as derived from different origins. There is an overlap of medical and non-medical issues. There is a remarkable amount of clear-cut origins in either one of the domains. Realizing this helps foster an adequate reaction, despite the lack of a common understanding of when and what. Usually, a highly individual exploration is inevitable in order to reach a point of certainty, which reaction might be helpful. While over-emphasizing the medical side of suffering leads to the pitfall of unjustified medicalization, with the consequence of potentially harmful or at least ineffective treatment, over-emphasizing of the existential side of suffering might lead to an empowerment for acceptance which will leave patients untreated despite adequate remedies available.

Medical Reflexes and Their "End of Life Care" Applicability

There are typical general medical attitudes and approaches towards end of life. Overcoming boundaries (Fighting death) describes the attitude of non-acceptance of approaching death. Treatment tends to be aggressive, all technical support systems are used and even a small likelihood of success is labeled as a chance not to be missed. This attitude is equally found among professionals and patients. Accepting limitations (Promoting Acceptance) in contrast, describes an attitude of letting go. The notion is that further aggressive treatment, or treatment at all, is not worth it anymore. The available medical treatment offers are not promising enough to try them. Again, this attitude can be found on both sides among professionals as well as among patients. Most commonly, we find a different feature; ambivalence, a mixture of the attitudes above, is realistically the most characteristic reaction. It describes, on the one hand, the change of attitudes over time from acceptance to fighting (and reverse) in sometimes very rapid cycles. On the other hand, it refers to simultaneously expressed contradictory wishes and expectations: "I wish it would be over soon" and "I want to live up to the marriage of my currently 6-year-old grandson" in one conversation is an example not rarely met. This ambivalence only appears irrational at a superficial first glance. It is neither a sign of weakness of patients and professionals, nor a sign of the ineffectiveness of intervention promoting understanding of the implications of the disease.

Ambivalence is a highly sophisticated cultural and emotional achievement. It is possibly one of the important differences between humans and animals. We are (for good or bad) able to predict and reflect on the effects of our deeds in the future. Ambivalence expresses humanity at its core. Therefore ambivalence earns respect and needs to be respected in general terms, as well as in the medical decision-making process. Respect for personal attitudes and belief is implicated in the palliative care approach. In general, ambivalence is not considered to be helpful in medical decision-making, as decisions like informed consent have to be documented in a legally resilient way. The medical approach usually does not like ambiguity or ambivalence, as it challenges the established procedure. This procedure is a logical step by step pathway. At the beginning, there is a pathological finding (diagnosis). Critical analysis and evaluation of these findings then lead to a treatment proposal as the second step. This is followed by the intervention, once consent is obtained. Then, as a fourth step, the result is evaluated. If the result is satisfactory, the treatment is continued until the treatment goal is reached; if the result is unsatisfactory treatment plans have to be reviewed and changed. This is generally true for every medical intervention, including palliative care interventions aimed at the relief of suffering. But, as said above, not all suffering derives from pathological findings. It carries aspects of existentiality, and expresses natural humanity in its origin. This leads to important questions regarding the medical reaction to suffering:

a)   Is medical treatment justified, if the underlying condition is not a pathological one?

b)   If there is no pathological finding, there is no good medical indication. If there is no real medical indication how does one deal with the medical options available?

c)   Some options are considered to be very helpful in end of life care, often supported by the strong wishes of the patient. Does this strong wish then potentially overrule the necessity of an indication?

d)   And if so, are there any limitations left to restrain wish-fulfilling medicine in end of life care? How about dying wishes in this context?

Relevant examples for questions like that in palliative care are frequent. How does one treat anxiety in a palliative care unit? Is the treatment to be abandoned to pharmacological treatment or is anxiety to be made bearable by emotional presence? Is it justified to pharmacologically treat existential distress? Is the unpleasant but possibly natural feeling of "fear in the face of death" to be made acceptable, or to be ended, possibly even including the act of killing or assisted suicide as ultimate ratio? Is suffering to be ended or to be made bearable?

Ideas for Tackling the Problem

There are no checklists ensuring escape from the possible pitfalls and how to make sure that misunderstandings are excluded. The key to a viable and stable therapeutic relationship in the context of existential suffering is based on the acknowledgment that we deal with unique individuals affected by life threatening diseases. This incorporates the ambivalence of aiming at removing all harmful influences medically, whenever possible, while still knowing that this does not reflect the whole story. Professionals in this field have to be courageous enough to allow their patients and themselves to meet on an emotional level that looks more deeply at the personal stories. Respectful understanding is a first step. Narratives, instead of checklists, help to classify medical options in the real lives of the humans affected. Professionals should try to pay respect to the person within the patient as well as to the patient within the person. No person is ever a patient without being a human with a unique biography, wishes, beliefs, hopes and fears. And, vice versa, almost every human being suffering from a disease and its consequences does have expectations, fears, hopes, experiences, successes and disappointments with the medical system. Characteristics of a successful professional respect-based relationship are honesty, emotional presence, empathy, reliability, competence, calmness, personal dedication, readiness for conflict and constant willingness to search.

Keeping these skills of a respect-based relationship in mind as a baseline for any communication, the concept of symptom control for suffering in palliative care, to avoid or to reduce discomfort as effectively as possible, comprises three major milestones: one is medical (somatic) interventions and psychosocial support. Second, is to accept the interpretation highness of the patient: "pain is when the patient says it hurts". Only what the patient considers to be important is really important. The third approach focuses on the non-medical dimension: there should be enough room for non-medical issues and approaches reflecting the existential side of the story. There should be space to emphasize the importance of being oneself with all conflicting and competing interests, perceptions, hopes and fears; and there should be enough security to offer a sheltered space for ambivalence. Then, the gap between medical and existential suffering might become bridgeable.

Bibliography

Bausewein, Claudia et al. (2016): EAPC white paper on outcome measurement in palliative care: Improving practice, attaining outcomes and delivering quality services – Recommendations from the European Association for Palliative Care (EAPC) Task Force on Outcome Measurement, in: Palliative Medicine 30, 1: 6-22. Online: http://assistenza.cottolengo.org/doc/ICare/Cure%20palliative%20valutazioni%20quantitative%20Pall%20Med%202016.pdf (last access 03/05/2019).

Cherny, Nathan I/Radbruch, Lukas/The Board of the European Association of Palliative Care (2009): European Association for Palliative Care (EAPC) recommended framework for the use of sedation in palliative care, in: Palliative Medicine 23, 7. Online: https://journals.sagepub.com/doi/pdf/10.1177/0269216309107024 (last access 03/05/2019).

Chochinov, Harvey M. (2012): Dignity therapy. Final words for final days, Oxford/New York: Oxford Univ. Press.

DGP (Deutsche Gesellschaft für Palliativmedizin) (2015): Leitlinien Palliativmedizin für Patienten mit einer nicht heilbaren Krebserkrankung, in: Leitlinienprogramm Onkologie. Online: https://www.awmf.org/uploads/tx_szleitlinien/128-001OL1_S3_Palliativmedizin_2015-07.pdf (last access 03/05/2019).

WHO: WHO Definition of Palliative Care. Online: http://www.who.int/cancer/palliative/definition/en (last access 03/05/2019).

Fig. 3.1: Maslow's Hierarchy of Needs. Source: Wikimedia Commons: https://commons.wikimedia.org/wiki/File:Mazlow%27s_Hierarchy_of_Needs.svg (CC BY-SA 3.0).

Suffering in the Context of Mental Illness

A Challenge for Ethics in Psychiatry

Gwendolin Wanderer

Suffering poses a challenge for bioethics in general and for ethics in psychiatry in particular; a challenge which at least by the latter has so far largely been evaded. This seems to be due to the subjectivity and the complexity of the matter of suffering. An understanding of suffering does not directly help to set up principles that guide actions, but is essential for an understanding of a patient's individual values or, in other words, for the spelling out of what, for him or her, constitutes a *good life*. Phenomenology carries out investigations of the lived experiences. In the context of bioethical issues, these phenomenological findings include the experiences of the persons involved in morally problematic situations: like vulnerability, authenticity, suffering or empathy. This contributes to a better understanding of how the main principles of bioethics could be applied. (Svenaeus 2020: 14 ff.)

The approach of *second-order empathy* suggests an empathic response to mental illness suffering that is informed by psychiatric expertise as well as by the findings of phenomenological and hermeneutical philosophy. It contributes to the reflection upon the virtuous psychiatrist, but has to be supplemented by social-ethical reflections. Often, professional, institutional or societal values and conditions are a source of suffering themselves, especially in the context of mental illness. In this text, the term suffering *in the context of mental illness* suggests that there are various kinds of suffering that could and should be considered apart from the suffering from illness symptoms. There are all sorts of sufferings in the closer or wider context of mental illness that can – and ought to be – distinguished.

This text intends to illustrate the significance of the aspect of suffering for ethics in psychiatry, as well as the challenges this implies.

The Opacity of Suffering – a Case Study

In order to envision the challenges that go along with the obligation to acknowledge and alleviate suffering in the psychiatric context, it might be helpful to take a look at an American case study that was published in the Journal of Medical Ethics some years ago (Schneider, Bramstedt 2005).

© BRILL SCHÖNINGH, 2022 | DOI:10.30965/9783657715428_005

The case study actually focussed on differing approaches to assessing a psychiatric patient's decision-making capacity (DMC). It depicted the coercive hospitalization of an 81-year-old man, who had been brought to a medical centre by the police (which he later referred to as the 'Gestapo') due to a generalized weakness. He had lived in his non-functioning motor vehicle together with his dog. A diagnosed profound microcytic anaemia needed to be medically treated. He had a scrotal hernia of the size of a football and possible dementia. Still, he disapproved of medical care. His records showed that he was a Second World War veteran and that he had been diagnosed with chronic paranoid schizophrenia many years ago, but never underwent psychiatric treatment. The patient himself denied all medical complaints except for chronic knee and leg pain. According to the psychiatrists, the patient lacked DMC. Since medical treatment was not urgently needed, and considering that the old man "did not demonstrate clearly delusional or inaccurate reasons for refusal of care, the psychiatrist argued that a court would likely not order compulsory treatment." (ibid). In the end, the patient was put in psychiatric detention due to grave disability and was transferred to a psychiatric unit for continued care.

> "[...] Ultimately he was transferred to a VA nursing home [VA = U.S. Department of Veteran Affairs (G.W.)] where he remained unhappy at losing his independence and his dog. He eloped several times from the nursing home and was found wandering the VA grounds by police. He was transferred to an inpatient psychiatry ward where permission was granted by his conservator for him to receive antipsychotic medication by injection, monthly. He had improvement in his overall level of paranoia and agitation but continued to refuse all other forms of medical treatment. More than two years after his initial presentation, he is still living in the VA nursing home, and has now asked for his hernia to be fixed." (ibid.)

The interventions seem to have been to the old man's beneficence. Still, since the case lacks a first-person perspective, there is a lot we do not get to know. We might wonder if the old man had originally *suffered* when residing in his car. He obviously had not complained about it. To him, the inconveniences caused by his homelessness and by his bodily ailments were perhaps secondary to some other kind of suffering. Since his DMC was obviously reduced – he was probably not able to make free choices, to calculate the possible danger of his lifestyle neither to himself nor to others – the obligation to medical care comes in, even in the absence of verbalized suffering. The man was distressed when he was being brought to the medical institution. The fact that he eloped from the care home he had been transferred to, hints to the fact that he probably disliked being there. He obviously missed his dog. But did that make him suffer? And even if it did, would it have been the better choice not to offer this somatically and mentally ill and homeless old man medical treatment and housing? His suffering might have decreased in the long run, after having adapted to the new situation.

We will never know what the old man in the depicted case study will have concluded or felt within the scope of his ability to conclude or feel. The question whether a patient eventually approved of his or her therapy or not in psychiatric contexts often remains unanswered. This gap is haunting, since one is left with a feeling of uncertainty concerning the moral quality of the decisions made. They might have been against the patient's values and could maybe have contributed to his or her suffering.

The case study illustrates that it is hardly possible to deduct clear standards for action from the quantity or quality of a person's suffering. Still, it will largely be accepted that suffering should, in some way, at least be acknowledged, if not alleviated. For medicine, the alleviation of suffering is even considered a primary aim. However, there is often just a vague understanding of what suffering actually is, and what physicians – and in our context: psychiatrists – could do to prevent or even alleviate it.

The Distinction of *Symptom* and *Suffering* and Its Specific Relevance in Psychiatry

For Eric Cassell, it was important to point to the fact that symptoms and suffering are distinct phenomena and that therefore the cure of disease and the alleviation of suffering are not to be equalled (Cassell 1983: 522). Symptoms with an identified cause that seem to be manageable and will cease may not necessarily cause suffering (Cassell 1983: 522).

In his texts on *The Nature of Suffering and the Goals of Medicine* Cassell suggests that it is *severe distress* associated with "events that threaten the intactness of the person" (Cassell 1982: 639, 2004:32) that equals the notion of suffering. He explicates that suffering occurs when for instance the illness-induced pain cannot be controlled, when its origin cannot be identified, when a patient is overpowered by his pain, when he becomes hopeless, suffers from reduced self-esteem because of the treatment's side-effects (like weight-gain or hair-loss) and is severely hindered in fulfilling the various roles in life and in pursuing personal goals. All these effects may threaten *the self, relations with others* and *relations with the surrounding world*, which according to Cassell constitute a *person*. (Cassell 2004: 33) An ignorance of such suffering might become a source of suffering itself. This, as Cassel puts it, contradicts the medical obligation to alleviate human suffering. The only way to avoid this 'paradox' would be to understand the medical obligation as a twin one: to cure disease and to acknowledge and alleviate suffering. (ibid.). In order to identify a patient's suffering he (or she) would have to be asked about it.[1]

Cassel's intention was to widen the medical gaze and motivate doctors to strive for a patient centered medicine. His focus, though, was obviously on somatic medicine, which is indicated by the fact that he considers the medical *cure* of *disease* to be one of the two medical obligations, not the therapy of *mental illness*. Since the boundaries between 'normal' mental states and pathological ones are still – and will probably always be – fuzzy, and since there might always remain some level of uncertainty about the definite identification, *mental disorder* or *mental illness* remain the preferred terms in the psychiatric literature.

Svenaeus (2018) and Holzhey-Kunz (2014) point to a specific of mental illness-suffering: In mental illness, the person seems to be threatened in the first place: affectivity, the self, cognitive ability, interpersonal skills and confidence of the self and of the future may be impaired (Svenaeus 2018)[2]. If these aspects become illness symptoms, the obligation to cure (or at least to relieve symptoms) and the obligation to acknowledge and alleviate suffering merge. According to Svenaeus, this conflation increases the risk that "comprehensible affects are likely to become subject to psychiatric treatment" (ibid) and is likely to lead to "medicalizing existential suffering" (ibid.). The comprehensible within the incomprehensible would, according to Svenaeus, have to be safeguarded. Whereas Holzhey-Kunz, in that respect, brings the hermeneutical approach of psychoanalysis into play, as a possibility to construe an underlying, subconscious meaning of the particular suffering, Svenaeus points to the importance of distinguishing between different kinds of suffering, like *illness-suffering, existential* and *political suffering*. According to Svenaeus, mental illness involves existential suffering in most cases, whereas in somatic illness existential suffering is involved merely in severe cases (Svenaeus 2018:8). He comes to the conclusion that mental illness is prone to medicalisation and

---

1   At the same time, Cassell also suggests that another person's suffering could also be observed, even measured, presupposed the observer has an "open view, empathy and experience". The experienced and empathetic doctor according to Cassell has the ability to share another person's experiences by imagining what it would be like to be in the same or in a similar situation. Braude notes that suffering generally encompasses more than medicine can acknowledge and should be able to attend to, and therefore criticizes Cassel for being too optimistic and rather uncritical about the possibility of a holistic gaze and the scope of medical means. (Braude 2012: 275)

2   In fact, Svenaeus states that mental disorders inevitably affect the personality or the self, and are not just ailments that patients *have*. (Svenaeus 2013: 1176) The symptoms and diagnosis listed in the DSM cannot be detected without judgements about *who* the patient is. (Ibid.)

draws attention to a diagnosis that considers the psychiatric patient's lifeworld in order to be better able to distinguish between illness-induced and other suffering, and with this joins the critics of the classification manuals of mental disorders. Descriptive phenomenology would help to better comprehend at what levels people suffer when they are affected by mental illness and what it means for them. This implies the ethical obligation to adequately acknowledge and alleviate it – within the realms of possibility and of the desirable.

Svenaeus, however, does not dwell on the obvious consequences for a responsible response to suffering that is either caused by an imbalanced metabolism, fundamental uncertainty concerning the individual existence, or societal conditions like stigmatization, distressing working conditions and the like. This, though, would well connect with an ethics of vulnerability (considering that suffering is the actuality of vulnerability) that distinguishes between ontological, structural and moral vulnerability. Whereas ontological vulnerability calls for care, counselling and comfort, structural and moral vulnerability rather call for moral action in solidarity e.g. with those who suffer due to disrespect or inequality. (See Haker 2019: 410 and 2021, within this volume.)

Due to its depth of intervention, psychopharmacological medication may also affect the self in such a way that dealing with existential suffering is hindered. Antidepressants may have the medical effect that the mood spectrum of the patients becomes richer and, in Svenaeus' words, "allows the self to become at home with itself and in the world" (Svenaeus 2015: 1180). At the same time, "the mood spectrum also becomes poorer in that the steep ups and downs of intense moods such as sadness and joy are cut off. The sine curve of life is characteristically flattened out by antidepressants, something that can be both praised and lamented by patients" (Ibid., 1180). The fact that patients might not recognize their new mood profile indicates that antidepressants not only help to alleviate suffering induced by mental disorder, but also have an effect on the self. Temperament and emotional dispositions are basic to personality (or selfhood). (Ibid., 1180)

This depth of intervention of psychotropic drugs illustrates that, in the context of psychiatry, the therapeutic intention to alleviate mental illness symptoms is prone to being a source of suffering itself. This shall be illustrated by a second case study.

Suffering from Passivity and Hopelessness – a Second Case Study

The first-person account of the former psychiatric patient Wilma Boevink (2015) illustrates several aspects of suffering that have been depicted above.

Here, Boevink reflects upon her hospitalization in a psychiatric institution and her decision to end medical therapy and instead turn to an alternate way to recovery. In the following excerpt, she recalls her experience with therapy.

> Looking back at those years, I guess my professional caregivers settled for the level of stability that 'they achieved for me'. For them I had come to a point where my life quality was acceptable in their eyes and so the main goal of their interventions was to prevent relapse and maintain status quo. They never asked me about my opinion, nor about my experienced quality of life. Had they done that, I would have told them that I was very scared of another psychotic episode, but that I never would settle for status quo. I was on enormous amounts of medication, my body weight was far too high, my hair curled from the medication, and other side effects like sedation kept me from functioning the way I wanted. Looking at pictures of myself from that time, I see a kind of Rubenesque Shirley Temple.
>
> But I wasn't asked about my opinion. Informed consent wasn't invented back then, and I doubt whether they would have thought that I was capable of understanding their information and give my consent to their decisions. Yes, I was scared to death of the next hell of psychosis. I came to a standstill and needed all my energy to survive, I blocked all my natural dynamics that come with life. I clung to a very low-profile daily routine of eating, drinking, resting and taking medication. 'She is not motivated to get well' was another professional judgment of my behavior back then. But I just couldn't permit myself anything new in my life. [...]
>
> What happened so that this hopeless situation is now behind me? Perhaps I would never have fought out of my prison of 'negative symptoms' if the medical approach to my situation was effective; but it wasn't. Although I took medication and followed psycho-education, which made me very compliant, my symptoms didn't ameliorate or disappear. About twice a year, I got into psychotic crisis. That kind of life was no longer acceptable for me. I'd rather die than to go on like that. In this dark period, I accidentally came across a first person account on recovery from severe distress. My desperation made me open to something new, to take the plunge – a kind of 'do it' or die – for a new way of experiencing my life. And slowly but surely I opened up to hope. Every day I gathered a little more courage to be curious enough about this new perspective. I got angry enough about my experiences as a 'hopeless case' in psychiatry to be ready for a hopeful and empowering perspective on what happened to me. It didn't end my suffering, but at least then I knew I should act. (Boevink 2015)

The author's first-person account of her psychopharmacological treatment and her decision to turn to the so called *recovery* approach, illustrates her multiple suffering. In the first place, she suffered from psychotic crisis twice a year and the rest of the time, she was "scared to death of the next hell of psychosis". Phenomenological studies contribute to a better insight into experiences in the context of suffering from psychotic disorder. A brief look at a list of symptoms and some brief phenomenological descriptions shall give us a glimpse at what it might have meant for the patient to be struck by a psychosis that was accompanied by destructive voices and which she describes as "hell".

Psychotic disorders like schizophrenia are qualified as *disorder of the self*, which means that those struck by such disorder suffer from a disturbance of their pre-reflective self-awareness. This is shown in the following list of symptoms in schizophrenia:

> Schizophrenia can include "[...] experiences of hyper-reflexivity and diminished self-affection, meaning that the flow of the pre-reflexive self is either intensified and interrupted in various ways or flattened out in feelings of non-existence [...]. Hyper-reflexivity will be experienced as a basic form of alienation of selfhood, the flow of experience being constantly interrupted by thoughts and voices which feel foreign in origin, leading to hallucinations (mainly auditory), delusions, and disorganized thoughts on part of the patient. Diminished self-affection is correlated with the so-called negative symptoms of schizophrenia, the patient feeling non-present and *anonymous*, unable to take initiatives and see the possibility of doing anything. Speech and communication in both cases are severely affected, leading to 'word-salad' and being cut off from contact with others" (DSM IV quoted in Svenaeus 2013: 1177)

If the basic belonging of one's stream of consciousness, the "flow of pre-reflexive self" is disturbed, the patient is alienated from his previous self. The ownership of his will, his thoughts and feelings, is threatened (see e.g. Ratcliffe 2008). The patient struggles to regain ownership and meaningfulness.

But then, Boevink also suffered from various side-effects of the psychotropic drugs she was given, and most from the effect that they kept her in a dull and passive state. She was neither able to take the initiative to actively participate in therapy, nor was she able to express how much she suffered from the reduced self-esteem due to her weight-gain and her altered hair structure. Finally, she suffered from being considered a "hopeless case". Psychotic disorders occur in recurrent attacks and then tend to become chronic. This is a challenge for the therapeutic team and most of all for the patients themselves.

Boevenik retrospectively thought that the doctors did probably not consider her to be capable of decision making, and consequently she was not included in therapy decisions. The empowerment-oriented *recovery* approach[3] helped

---

3 Alternative strategies to *recovery* are strategies that intend to empower mentally disordered persons to better cope with their symptoms without or accompanied by psychotropic medication. The so called *recovery movement* is part of a post psychiatric approach. Post psychiatry acknowledges a pluralism of medical (and psychological) approaches to mental illness, but claims that "the non-technical aspects of mental health problems should have priority over the technical aspects" (Bracken/Thomas 2015: 137) and suggests a "collaboration between service users and professionals" (ibid.).

her to regain agency and to learn how to better cope with the threatening destructive voices who wanted her to kill herself in the course of psychotic crises, which was an "endless struggle" though. This alternative path to *recovery* did not end but at least alleviate her suffering, since it made her feel less passive and probably more connected to *who she is*.

The aspect of *ownership* might be of special importance for patients with psychotic disorder, but it may also be of importance for patients who suffer from other mental illnesses. For some patients it may be important to understand the experienced symptoms as appendant to one's *self*. Strategies to cope with the symptoms interfuse with one's personality. Or, in other words, there can be a sense of "ownership" of the suffering which is of relevance to the sufferer. "Pragmatically, owning one's fate can feel more important than enjoying it." (Mann 1992: 545) Understanding the meaning of suffering that is owned or even self-induced by a patient can help to therapize it. This connects with psychodynamic theories and exceeds biologic psychiatry. Psychodynamics attempts to interpret mental states in terms of unconscious innate forces and in terms of conscious decisions.

According to Mann, deliberate suffering can for example be observed when dependant relationships are being replaced by addictive substances or other habitual behaviour, like binge eating, that seem more controllable than relationships or bad feelings. The deliberate habitual suffering can be the more sufferable choice when compared to uncontrollable suffering. According to Mann, this is a possible starting point for empowerment, a struggle to become aware of and regain ownership. For some, this may be an alternative, better way of coping with their illness than undertaking a longstanding psychopharmacological therapy. For others, it is important to know that the symptoms are merely illness-induced and not part of their person. They might suffer less from submitting themselves to psychiatric institutions.

Suffering as a Decisive Aspect of Personhood and Autonomy

As depicted above, uncontrollable and overpowering pain, pain of unidentifiable origin, reduced self-esteem, hopelessness and hindrance in fulfilling personal life-goals according to Cassell trigger suffering. Suffering is conceived by him as something that exceeds illness-symptoms such as pain (and also nausea, breathlessness and giddiness). As has been amended, in mental illness, symptoms and the threatening of the person mostly coincide. This has consequences for the psychiatrist, whose obligation is to cure the patient (or at least to relieve his symptoms) and *at the same time* to acknowledge and alleviate the patient's suffering. Although, he has to be careful not to medicalize the individual patient's attempt to make sense of her pain and to develop an attitude towards her suffering. Medical means might be adequate to get symptoms under control, but not to deal with the active struggling of the individual *person* with the threats of mental disorder symptoms – even if this active struggling is in itself distorted. This definitely challenges psychiatry as well as ethics in psychiatry, since the struggle for an adequate response to mental illness suffering is also an ethical question, and since *personhood* is also a normative term.

According to Stanghellini and Rosefort (2015), a hermeneutical phenomenological approach to personhood "combines phenomenological findings on the experiential features of being a self with an explanatory framework that takes into account both the voluntary and involuntary features of human existence." (319 f.) Within this phenomenologically informed hermeneutical philosophy, the complexity of the notions of *human being, selfhood* and *personhood* can be assessed and investigated. Whereas phenomenology contributes to an understanding of the descriptive notions of human being (in distinction to animals) and selfhood (e.g. the phenomenological structures of human subjectivity), the notion of personhood is a normative notion. "To be a person may be a fact, but it is also a task" (320), Stanghellini and Rosefort explain, with reference to the French philosopher Paul Ricoeur. A person is "what we are and who we want to become. To be a human being is to be a person, and yet we care about being a (certain kind of) person." (320) On the one hand, there is the normative aspect of personhood; our striving to be a certain kind of person. On the other hand, in becoming the person that we want to become, we are continuously challenged by some otherness. This creates a tension, sometimes even a conflict "between otherness and selfhood in being a person over time." (Ibid.)

This otherness, that challenges our identity (or *self*, the terms are being used interchangeably), consists of aspects of our existence that are beyond our control, like the encounter with other people and the world, as well as bodily processes, like ageing or being struck by illness. The tension between otherness and selfhood can be difficult to cope with.

> "My body changes, becomes different as the years go by, and I may become alienated by these transformations. I can accept such changes, despair because of them, or fight them, but every one of those attitudes affects the person that I am. In short, to be a person involves the inescapable struggle with the otherness that constitutes the person that I am." (320)

In the second case study within this text, the patient suffered from a pharmacological medication-induced body-transformation, most of all from her weight gain and her hair looking different than before. Sedation kept her from functioning the way she wanted. The patient was confronted with an otherness that conflicted with her identity. She did not manage to reinterpret this new body image and her lack of drive as a part of herself.

Hermeneutic phenomenology emphasizes the "interpretive character of being human." (321) This means, that human beings are constantly challenged to reinterpret in what way they still are the peculiar being that they think that they are and intend to be.

This pre-reflexive experience of ownership and agency, the experience that *it is me who experiences*, is "a necessary but not an exhaustive part of my experience of being who and what I am." (327) The experience of being a self in the world also involves "temporality in the sense that I not only care about who I am now, but also, who I was and who I want to be". (327)

Even though the sense of ownership and agency as well as the perception of temporality can be distorted in pathologies of the self or of affect, this interpretive character of being human does not come to a halt. According to Rosfort (2019), the notion of personhood is vital to phenomenological psychopathology, especially when the attempt to make sense of the alienating aspect of mental illness is concerned. "The disturbance of self-awareness involved in mental illness often entails a sense of alienation and unbearable passivity." (Ibid. 340) Rosford contrasts this view with Paul Ricoeur's notion of suffering as "the most vivid forms of self-consciousness." (340 f.)

At that point, Rosfort especially follows Minkowski (1999), who argues that we "engage with our suffering and with the world through suffering" and "are searching for the meaning(s) of our suffering". (Ibid.) But suffering can also be so unbearable that a patient's sense of self can become "so dramatically disturbed that his identity is submerged in an anonymous and alienating process of painful otherness" (341).[4] Pain can be "so excruciating that the experience is completely drained of thought and reflection. But in the afterglow of pain, thought re-emerges. We do something with what we feel. We relate ourselves to our feelings, or as Karl Jaspers (1997) argues, we always position ourselves to our suffering." (ibid. 341) Often, we learn from retrospective first-person accounts in what way a patient suffered.

The aspect that is the most challenging about personhood is, in how far it is supposed to comprise a notion of autonomy that differs from the capability

---

4   A mental health care professional could, as Rosfort suggests, help the patient to narratively reconfigure his suffering structured around the notion of personhood in order to "appropriate his pain and make the otherness part of who he is". Also, such a narrative approach could also help the health care professional to recognize the patient as a person. (342)

based aspect of informed consent. According to the elaborations above, suffering is individual. As such, one might say, it is an expression of autonomy. Such suffering cannot be assessed with pragmatic measures of meaning. "Suffering is the expression of an individuality that we can make sense of only by paying attention to the unique tension of voluntary and involuntary that makes each and every one of us the person that he or she is." (Stanghellini/Rosfort, ibid: 330) The most important aspect of the principle of autonomy in the clinical context is, that it safeguards "the individual character of the patient's suffering against heteronomous tendencies at work in all therapeutic models." (331)

> "Besides being a normative principle, autonomy is an experiential fact and an existential problem that is dramatically expressed in mental illness. Hermeneutical phenomenology shows that autonomy is not merely a general ethical principle applied to therapy, but an integral part of the suffering of mental illnesses. [... I]n suffering we are dealing with a struggle of and for autonomy." (331)

This struggle is the attempt to make sense of the unbearable passivity involved in suffering. Whereas the notion of misery emphasizes the paralyzing passivity of pain, the notion of suffering emphasizes an active engagement that makes our suffering personal.

According to Stanghellini and Rosfort "[... d]istinguishing suffering and misery is fundamental to phenomenological psychopathology because it allows both the patients and the mental health-care professionals to recognize the patient as an autonomous person" (ibid.).

First- and Second-order Empathy

It has become sufficiently clear that to acknowledge and alleviate suffering in the context of mental illness is a comprehensive task. *Empathy*, which can be defined as an ability to share another person's experiences by imagining what it would be like to be in the same or in a similar situation, can be seen as a prerequisite for the acknowledgement of suffering.

An *experienced doctor* would be able to identify and, at least to some extent, understand a patient's suffering, Cassell (2004) suggested, as was already mentioned earlier. However, the above elaborations have illustrated that this is quite challenging, since the experience of patients with mental disorder, especially with psychotic symptoms, often significantly differs from 'normal' experience. Therefore, Fuchs (2013), on the basis of and in contrast to Karl Jasper's notion on the incomprehensibility of psychotic experience, introduced a "second-order-empathy" as a method to adequately comprehend and react to psychotic experiences.

> "Severe aberrations of experience such as those that can be met with in schizophrenia would seem to require a different, and more theoretical kind of empathy. [U]nderstanding psychotic experiences like schizophrenic, melancholic, or manic ones requires a kind of training that goes beyond a phenomenological conception of spontaneous nonconative empathic skills, and at the same time avoids the pitfalls of conative empathy based on the clinician's personal experiences and common sense categories. The achievement of this training can be named second-order-empathy." (Ibid.: 342)

According to Fuchs, to achieve second-order empathy is a complex process. It necessarily includes an acknowledgement of the other person's autonomy and consequently an acknowledgement of the fact that the other person's life-world differs from one's own. Also, according to Fuchs it is necessary to "neutralize [... one's] natural attitude [...] to understand the other's experience as if it took place in a world like [... one's] own." The "existential structures of the world the other lives in" need to be reconstructed (e.g. detorted perception of temporality). Then one may "attempt to understand the other's experience as meaningfully situated in a world that is indeed similar to [... one's] own but also indelibly marked by the other person's particular existence, and by that person's endeavour to become who she or he is." (342 f.)

> "Achieving second-order empathy thus requires me to set aside my own prereflexive, natural attitude (in which my first-order empathic capacities are rooted), and to approach the other's world as I would do while exploring an unknown and alien country." (343)

A critical note to this second-order empathy approach concerns the method: According to Rashed (2015:8) "[... t]he psychopathologists rightly saw the problem to be one of privation of meaning rather than its intrinsic absence, but were wrong to introduce a problematic method to seek that understanding [...]"[5]. As human beings, we are always 'in the world'. *Bracketing natural world-life*, therefore seems difficult, if not impossible. (Ibid.) Apart from this, the author doubts that "an attitude which emphasizes differences is the right one to adopt" (ibid.: 14). To see obscure differences would have a stigmatizing and de-humanizing effect, even though the approach of second-order empathy intends to protect psychotic patients from the de-humanizing position of

---

5 A Husserlian *phenomenological reduction* to which the concept of second-order-empathy refers, according to Rashed neglects the world's opacity and indeterminacy (ibid.: 11).

lying outside the realms of meaning. (Ibid.) The image of the 'unknown and alien country that is being explored' seems to neglect the aspect of the perception of a 'shared space', shared values and beliefs. It also seems to lack another decisive aspect: the aspect of *care*. Haker notes that "the responsible response to a suffering person is not a self-centered or world-exploring experience but a response to an other whom one *cares* about" (Haker 2022: 129). In order for it to be an experience of sympathy, perception and concern for the other must converge. (Ibid.)

Notwithstanding these critical notes, one may agree with Fuchs that subject-oriented approaches to psychiatric diagnosis and classification are strongly needed in order to pursue, among others, the goal "[...] to reopen and enrich [a] methodically guided understanding of the patient's subjective experience [...] to prepare the ground for psychotherapy as a hermeneutic re-interpretation of meanings, motives and strivings [...]" and "[...] to maintain the connections of psychiatry to the social sciences and the humanities with their longstanding tradition of understanding the human mind." (Fuchs 2010:273) The spectrum of the patient's subjective experience includes the aspect of suffering as a struggle to regain meaning, ownership and agency.

We do not know whether the attitude of second-order empathy would have led to different decisions on the side of the care-givers in the given case-studies. The psychiatrists and ethicists involved in the therapy decisions of the aged mentally ill veteran would probably also have recommended compulsory hospitalization and treatment. Or would they have thought of ways to allow the old man to see his dogs or even to find alternative housing for him? Would they have considered ambulant treatment on the basis of a better understanding of the patient's individual way of life? At least, there might have been a better perception of the diminished first-person perspective.

As far as the second case study is concerned, one might speculate that first- or second-order empathy would probably have enabled a less dissymmetrical encounter with the psychiatric professionals.

> "The phenomenological perspective opens up possibilities to understand the clinical encounter as a meeting with a suffering person and not only as a scientific investigation of the diseases of his body. In cases that concern the implementation of medical technologies, in addition to the face-to-face encounter, questions regarding reification or even instrumentalization of patients and their bodies will come to the fore." (Svenaeus 2020, ibid: 14)

On the one hand, Svenaeus' statement explicates implications of Fuchs' empathy approach. An openness to approaches to mental illness beyond the scientific ones is part of the second-order empathy. On the other hand, Svenaeus also goes even further when he states that the phenomenological view would identify reification and instrumentalization of patients and their bodies. Reification and instrumentalization are themselves threats to the integrity of the person, to their autonomy and their dignity. The empathic reaction to envisioned suffering would, therefore, also have to include an awareness of problematical values including a predominance of a certain approach to mental illness that side-lines other approaches. An empathic approach to suffering in psychiatry that includes phenomenologically informed perception and care would also have to encompass a motivation to further an ethical reflection of structures within psychiatric institutions and within society that are likely to cause suffering. Further social ethical reflection may supplement second-order empathy.

Summary and Conclusion

In the course of this text it has become apparent that suffering in the context of mental illness in some ways does not and in others does decisively differ from somatic illness suffering. Due to the fact that in mental illness comprehensible facets of existential and other forms of suffering may become illness symptoms, the obligation to cure (or at least to relieve symptoms) and the obligation to acknowledge and alleviate suffering merge. This conflation is likely to lead to medicalising existential and political suffering, which is problematic since this 1.) affects the patients' core personhood and 2.) shifts responsibility. To deal with the threats of mental disorder symptoms is an active struggle that cannot adequately be replaced by medical means. This struggling to reinterpret one's identity in the face of voluntary and involuntary otherness can be seen as an aspect of autonomy or rather as the core of subjectivity. The tension between one's identity and this otherness can be difficult to cope with. Counselling and empowerment strategies to regain agency or at least to regain rudimentary interpretive sovereignty over one's own suffering can sometimes be of greater help than medical means. This, along with the aspects of opacity and silence of suffering may hint psychiatrists to adopt an attitude of attentiveness and modesty. The method of second-order empathy intends to contribute to a subject-oriented approach to psychiatric diagnosis and classification. The perception and consideration of the patients' subjective suffering-experience offer interesting suggestions for ethics in psychiatry.

A responsible reaction to suffering, though, necessarily has to include the aspect of care which does not seem to be explicitly considered in second-order empathy.

To care for the sufferers in the context of mental illness means to care for different kinds of suffering that ought to be distinguished: suffering from symptoms, existential suffering, suffering from stigmatization, denied recognition, loss and other hardships. An adequate response to suffering in the context of mental illness, therefore, also has to reflect upon professional, institutional or societal values and conditions that may be a source of suffering themselves. In this text, this aspect was only briefly outlined but would be worth of further consideration.

To conclude, we can say that the quality and quantity of suffering does not allow a deduction of clear standards for action. Still, suffering can be considered as a key concept for ethics in psychiatry since it well illustrates the challenge of a subject-centred psychiatry and its ethical reflection.

Bibliography

American Psychoatric Association (2009): Diagnostic and statistical manual of mental disorders. DSM-IV-TR. 4. ed., text revision, Arlington, VA: American Psychiatric Assoc.

Bracken, Pat; Thomas, Philip (2015): Challenges to the Modernist Identity of Psychiatry: User Empowerment and Recovery, in John Z. Sadler, et al. (Eds.): The Oxford handbook of philosophy and psychiatry, Oxford: Oxford University Press (International perspectives in philosophy and psychiatry), 123-138.

Braude, Hillel (2012): Affecting the Body and Transforming Desire: The Treatment of Suffering as the End of Medicine, in *Philosophy, Psychiatry, & Psychology* 19: 265-278.

Boevink, Wilma (2015): Risk and Recovery: First-Person Account of Ethics in Relation to Recovery from Mental Illness, in: J.Z. Sadler/ C.W. van Staden/ K.W.M. Fulford: Psychiatric Ethics, Vol. 1, Oxford, 94-97.

Cassell, Eric J. (1982): The Nature of Suffering and the Goals of Medicine, in: *The New England Journal of Medicine:* 306, 639-645.

Cassell, Eric J. (2004): The Nature of Suffering and the Goals of Medicine, Second Edition, Oxford.

Connolly, William E. (1996): Suffering, Justice, and the Politics of Becoming, in: Culture, Medicine and Psychiatry 20: 251-277.

Fuchs, Thomas (2010): Subjectivity and Intersubjectivity in Psychiatric Diagnosis, in: Psychopathology 2010; 43:268-274.

Fuchs, Thomas (2013): The Phenomenology of Affectivity, in John Z. Sadler, et al. (Eds.): The Oxford handbook of philosophy and psychiatry, Oxford: Oxford University Press (International perspectives in philosophy and psychiatry), 612-631.

Haker, Hille (2019): Vulnerable Agency – Human Dignity and Gendered Violence. In: J. Rothschildt, Petrusek, M. (eds.): Dignity and Conflict: Contemporary Interfaith Dialogue on the Value and Vulnerability of Human Life. Notre Dame (University of Notre Dame Press), 2018, 393-436.

Haker, Hille (2022): Uprooted – Towards a Medical Ethics of Suffering, in Christof Mandry (Ed.): Suffering in theology and medical ethics, Paderborn, 113-144.

Hoffmaster, Barry (2014): Understanding Suffering, in: Green, Ronald M.; Palpant, Nathan J.: Suffering and Bioethics, Oxford/ New York, 31-53.

Holzhey-Kunz, Alice (2014): Phänomenologie oder Hermeneutik seelischen Leidens? In Thomas Fuchs, et al. (Eds.): Das leidende Subjekt. Phänomenologie als Wissenschaft der Psyche. Originalausgabe. Freiburg/ München: Verlag Karl Alber (Schriftenreihe der Deutschen Gesellschaft für Phänomenologische Anthropologie, Psychiatrie und Psychotherapie (DGAP), Band 3), 33-51.

Jaspers, Karl (1997): General Psychopathology (7th edn), J. Hoenig, M.W. Hamilton, trans., Baltimore MD.

Mann, David W. (1992): Psychiatric Pain and Deliberate Suffering, in: Psychoanalytic Dialogues 4: 545-560.

Marino, Gordon D.; Marino, Susan E. (2014): Paying Homage to the Silence of Suffering, in: Green, Ronald M.; Palpant, Nathan J.: Suffering and Bioethics, Oxford/ New York, 54-60.

Rashed, Mohammed Abouelleil (2015): *A Critical Perspective on Second-Order Empathy in Understanding Psychopathology: Phenomenology & Ethics. Theoretical Medicine and Bioethics* 36: 97-116v.

Radden, Jennifer (1988): Choosing to refuse. Patients' Rights and Psychotropic Medication, in: Bioethics 2 (2), 93-103.

Radden, Jennifer (2002): Psychiatric Ethics. Background Briefing. In *Bioethics: official journal of the International Association of Bioethics* 16 (5), pp. 397-411.

Radden, Jennifer (2009): Emotional Pain and Psychiatry, in: Moody Minds Distempered. Essays on Melancholy and Depression, Oxford/New York 2009, 111-129.

Ratcliffe, Matthew (2008): Feelings of Being. Phenomenology, Psychiatry and the Sense of Reality, Oxford.

Ratcliffe, Matthew (2015): Depression and the Phenomenology of Free Will, in John Z. Sadler, et al. (Eds.): The Oxford handbook of philosophy and psychiatry, Oxford: Oxford University Press (International perspectives in philosophy and psychiatry), 574-591.

Rosfort, René (2019): Personhood, in: G. Stanghellini et. Al.: The Oxford Handbook of Phenomenological Psychopathology, Oxford 335-343.

Stanghellini, Giovanni; Rosfort, René (2013): Empathy as a Sense of Autonomy, in: Psychopathology 46:337-344.

Stanghellini, Giovanni; Rosfort, René (2015): The Patient as an autonomous Person: Hermeneutical Phenomenology as a Resource for an Ethics of Psychiatrists, in: J.Z. Sadler/ C.W. van Staden/ K.W.M. Fulford: Psychiatric Ethics, Vol. 1, Oxford, 319-335.

Svenaeus, Fredrik (2017): Phenomenological Bioethics, London: Routledge.

Svenaeus, Fredrik (2014): The phenomenology of suffering in medicine and bioethics. In *Theoretical medicine and bioethics* 35: 407-420. DOI: 10.1007/s11017-014-9315-3.

Svenaeus, Fredrik (2015): Psychopharmacology and the Self, in John Z. Sadler, et al. (Eds.): The Oxford handbook of philosophy and psychiatry, Oxford: Oxford University Press (International perspectives in philosophy and psychiatry), 1171-1184.

Svenaeus, Fredrik (2018): Human Suffering and Psychiatric Diagnosis, in *Bioethica Forum* 11: 4-10.

Tellenbach, Hubertus (1974): Melancholie. Problemgeschichte, Endogenität, Typologie, Pathogenese, Klinik, Berlin/Heidelberg/New York (2nd ed.)

Wakefield, J. C. (1992). Disorder as harmful dysfunction: A conceptual critique of DSM-III-R's definition of mental disorder. *Psychological Review*, 99(2), 232-247. https://doi.org/10.1037/0033-295X.99.2.232, https://psycnet.apa.org/record/1992-27354-001 (accessed May 2019)

Zahavi, Dan (2005): Subjectivity and Selfhood. Investigating the First Person Perspective, Cambridge.

PART II

Suffering in the Medical-Ethical Discourse:
An Uncomfortable Concept

The Argument of "Suffering" in Opinions of the German Ethics Council (2007-2016)

Michael Coors

In 2007 the Ethics Council Act was passed by the German parliament. It defines the German Ethics Council as an independent committee of experts pursuing "the questions of ethics, society, science, medicine and law that arise and the probable consequences for the individual and society that result in connection with research and development, in particular in the field of the life sciences and their application to humanity" (EthRG 2,1). Its members are appointed by the president of the German Bundestag. They are experts in ethics, philosophy, theology, and medicine, and representatives of important groups in society (e.g. the Christian Churches and other religious communities). Publishing opinions on current ethical issues, especially in the life sciences is one of the tasks of the German Ethics Council. Between 2007 and 2016 it has published 13 opinions on various issues.

Opinions of the German Ethics Council (2009-2016)[1]
- *Anonymous relinquishment* of infants: tackling the problem (2009)
- Human *biobanks* for research (2010)
- Medical *benefits and costs* in healthcare: The normative role of their evaluation (2011)
- Preimplantation genetic diagnosis (*PGD*) (2011)
- *Human–animal mixtures* in research (2011)
- *Intersexuality* (2012)
- *Dementia* and self-determination (2012)
- The future of *genetic diagnosis* – from research to clinical practice (2013)

---

1   The short titles referred to below are printed in italics. All opinions are originally published in German and are translated into English. The page numbers refer to the German texts. The German texts of all opinions can be found on https://www.ethikrat.org/publikationen/kategorie/stellungnahmen, the English translations on https://www.ethikrat.org/en/publications/kategorie/opinions/?cookieLevel=not-set&cHash=d3866676809c124ade957d941894 27d2.

- *Biosecurity* – Freedom and Responsibility of Research (2014)
- *Incest* Prohibition (2014)
- *Brain Death* and decisions regarding organ donation (2015)
- *Embryo Donation*, Embryo Adoption and Parental Responsibility (2016)
- *Patient Welfare* as Ethical Standard for Hospitals (2016)

These opinions do not form a coherent canon of texts; the group of authors differs as the members of the Ethics Council have changed during the years. They deal with very different topics, and they do not aim to present a coherent ethical approach. Therefore, one cannot expect to find a unified concept of suffering in these texts. They are an interesting subject for ethical research nonetheless, precisely because they do not systematically reflect on how to use the concept of suffering. Thus, studying the way this term is used in the opinions might at least offer some insight into how ethic-experts use the concept of suffering as an argument in ethical debates.

Word-Statistics

The first step in analyzing how "suffering" is used as an argument in the opinions of the German Ethics Council is looking for how often the word is used. Table 1 shows that the usage varies enormously; from no usage of the word at all to 34 findings in the opinion on intersexuality. There are at least three opinions using the word "suffering" ("Leid/Leiden") or the verb "to suffer" ("leiden") more often than the other ones; these are the opinions on intersexuality, on human-animal mixtures[2], and on preimplantation genetic diagnosis (PGD).

---

2 The term "human-animal mixtures" is used as an umbrella term for interspecies chimeras and interspecies hybrids: "These are living organisms which include both human and animal material in different (albeit sometimes only small) proportions" (Deutscher Ethikrat 2011c, 13).

Table 5.1 Statistic on the use of "suffering/to suffer" and other words indicating vulnerabilities. All statistics are based on the German texts.

opinion	suffering	damage	need	impairment	pain
Intersexuality	34	21	5	17	5
Human-Animal Mixtures	27	13	1	4	17
PGD	15	9	5	19	1
Benefits and Costs	7	8	2	1	5
Dementia	6	6	2	8	4
Genetic diagnosis	6	4	1	31	1
Brain death	3	3	0	4	21
Anonymous relinquishment	3	7	27	7	0
Embryo Donation	3	5	0	3	0
Patient welfare	2	8	1	5	2
Incest	1	5	2	5	0
Biosecurity	0	0	0	3	0
Biobanks	0	139	0	13	3
Total	107	228	46	120	59

The word "suffering", though, is just one of many words indicating negative effects on persons. Other words used are "harm/damage" ("Schaden" in German), "pain" ("Schmerz"), "impairment" ("Beeinträchtigung") or "need/distress" ("Not"). One can summarize these terms as *phenomena of vulnerability* (on the concept of vulnerability cf. Mackenzie et al. 2014; Tham et al. 2014).

Some opinions do make use of some of these terms more extensively than others. For example, the paper on genetic diagnosis does very often use the word "impairment", because impairments due to genetic mutations are a crucial issue. The paper on the anonymous relinquishment of infants very often refers to the need or distress ("Not") a pregnant women might suffer from. To a large extend, the words used seem to depend on the topics discussed and on words typically used in the discourses the opinion-papers refer to.

The German term "Schaden" ("damage" or "harm" in English) is most often used in the opinion on biobanks, but in most cases in a clearly judicial sense. Nonetheless, these findings encourage taking a closer look at the difference between using the word "suffering" and using the other words listed above.

"Suffering" as an Argument?

I suggest distinguishing between at least four different ways of how "suffering/
to suffer" is used in the opinions of the German Ethics Council (A-D):

A: The verb "to suffer" is often used idiomatically, as in "suffering from an
illness" or "suffering from dementia" ("an einer Krankheit leiden", "an Demenz
leiden") without any emphasis on "suffering". In most of these cases, "to suffer"
can be replaced with hardly any loss of meaning; someone suffering from an
illness simply has an illness. These uses of "to suffer" are more or less ethically
irrelevant. This applies to 26 of the 107 findings of "suffering" in the opinions of
the German Ethics Council.[3]

B: Most often versions of "suffering/to suffer" are used explicitly or implicitly by reference to a moral principle of care, that is interpreted as a principle of avoiding and alleviating suffering. Reference to a principle of avoiding
suffering is, for example, made in the opinions on intersexuality (Deutscher
Ethikrat 2012a, 98;102), on dementia (Deutscher Ethikrat 2012b, 67) and on
human-animal mixtures (Deutscher Ethikrat 2011c, 48;56;63;69;109). In most
cases the opinions do not only refer to the moral principle of not doing harm
to someone – as is the case with Beauchamp and Childress' principle of non-
maleficence (Beauchamp/Childress 2013, 150) – but to an obligation to alleviate suffering, as in the opinions on Costs and Benefits (Deutscher Ethikrat
2011a, 12), intersexuality (Deutscher Ethikrat 2012a, 98;102;115), human-animal
mixtures (Deutscher Ethikrat 2011c, 63;109), embryo donation (Deutscher
Ethikrat 2016a, 90;122), brain death (Deutscher Ethikrat 2015, 99;110), patient
welfare (Deutscher Ethikrat 2016b, 68) and PGD (Deutscher Ethikrat 2011b,
146). In the opinion on intersexuality, the principle of avoiding suffering and
harm ("Prinzip der Leidens- und Schadensvermeidung") is introduced as an
interpretation of the principle of care ("Fürsorgeprinzip") (Deutscher Ethikrat
2012a, 106;109f.); to be obliged to care for someone means to be obliged to avoid
causing the suffering of this person.

This use of "suffering" or "to suffer" is certainly at the center of a moral use
of "suffering". Therefore, suffering comes ethically into view as something
to be avoided, and human actions have to take this principle of avoiding

---

3   For an overview see Tab. 2.

or alleviating suffering into account. To recognize that someone is suffering therefore implies prima facie a moral duty to help this person somehow. Accordingly, this use of "suffering" is the most frequent one in the opinions of the German Ethics Council. I counted 39 of 107 findings.

C: The third way versions of "suffering/to suffer" are used is related to the second use. While the second use focuses on suffering as something to be alleviated, the third use focuses on the suffering itself; it is what I call an existential use of the term, focusing on the fact that a person does suffer from something. This way of using the term suffering was found mainly in the opinions on intersexuality and on PGD. The first refers to the suffering of intersexual persons (Deutscher Ethikrat 2012a, 16;19;94;96;103;172;176), especially caused by medical action (Ibid., 19;103-105;165f.), and about their psychological and social suffering (Ibid., 152f.;165). The opinion on PGD refers to parents suffering under the burden of a heavily disabled child (Deutscher Ethikrat 2011b, 101;144;149) and to the possible suffering of a future child with a genetically caused disability (Ibid., 60;93;137;149). These sufferings are mentioned because the reader should understand them as a burden that has to be avoided. Thus, we are dealing with appeals to our moral duty to alleviate suffering, which connects these uses of "suffering" with the ones from category B. Yet, the focus here is not so much on the obligation the suffering implies for others, but rather on its impact on the life of the suffering person. I counted 35 findings of this use in the opinions.

D: A fourth way the word "suffering/to suffer" is used refers to the question of moral status. To be capable of suffering and feeling can be understood as an indicator for the moral status of living beings – an ethical tradition going back to Bentham (Bentham 1876). In regard to beings capable of suffering there exists a moral duty to avoid suffering. Hence, the question by which means we ascribe this capability of suffering to living beings becomes a crucial ethical question. This discussion on a pathocentric foundation of ethics is crucial to the question of animal rights. Accordingly, this use of "suffering" is to be found in the opinion-paper on human-animal mixtures in research – though, even here it is only explicitly focused upon six times (Deutscher Ethikrat 2011c, 36;63f.). It lays the basis, though, for how the reference to the moral principle to avoid harm and suffering is made in this paper and therefore has a crucial function. Throughout all the opinion papers, I found this use of "suffering" only seven times. The seventh finding is a short remark on the moral status of persons in the opinion-paper on organ transplantation and brain death (Deutscher Ethikrat 2015, 62).

Table 5.2   Overview on different ways of using the argument of suffering. A: idiomatic use; B: reference to the principle of avoiding and alleviating suffering; C: existential suffering; D: concerning the question of moral status.

opinion of the German Ethics Council	Total	A	B	C	D
Intersexuality	34	6	8	20	-
Human-Animal Mixtures	27	1	18	2	6
PGD	15	3	3	9	-
Benefits and Costs	7	4	3	-	-
Dementia	6	1	1	4	-
Genetic diagnosis	6	5	1	-	-
Brain death	3	-	2	-	1
Anonymous relinquishment	3	3	-	-	-
Embryo Donation	3	1	2	-	-
Patient welfare	2	1	1	-	-
Incest	1	1	-	-	-
Biosecurity	0	-	-	-	-
Biobanks	0	-	-	-	-
Total	107	26	39	35	7

Considering these findings, it seems plausible to argue that the term "suffering" finds its way into the opinions of the German Ethics Council by reference to the principle of care, which is interpreted as the principle of avoiding harm *and suffering*. It is this moral principle by which ethics is confronted with the concept of suffering. Because suffering is to be avoided or alleviated, the existential suffering of persons comes into view. Therefore, the focus of the following considerations will be on these two uses (B and C).

Due to the focus on the alleviation of suffering, suffering is primarily discussed as something *to be avoided*. There is little space left for the contrary question of how to accept certain forms of suffering as an implication of life (e.g. Schmidt 2011, 83-111; Liebsch 2014). Accordingly, by means of this focus it remains an open question here, whether the principle to avoid suffering implies that all suffering has to be avoided, or whether there is suffering we need to accept as part of being vulnerable persons. Nonetheless, the opinions of the German Ethics council do acknowledge that not all suffering can be avoided or alleviated (Deutscher Ethikrat 2012a, 102).

Who Suffers under Whom and from What?

My main argument so far has been that suffering becomes a topic of the ethical considerations in the opinions of the German Ethics Council due to the reference to the principle of care, which is interpreted as the obligation to avoid and alleviate suffering. I will now take a closer look at the argumentative uses of suffering in categories B and C.

The Principle of Care: Who is Obliged to Avoid Whose Suffering?

As would be expected, the opinions refer to the obligation (especially of physicians and researchers) to avoid or alleviate the suffering of patients with various illnesses, or of people who suffer from being without a child of their own. This obligation does not only refer to physicians, though, but also to society as a whole, as can be emphasized in regard to the German healthcare system based on solidarity (Deutscher Ethikrat 2011a, 12). Also, parents of future children might act under the obligation to avoid suffering of their future child, as is argued in the context of PGD (Deutscher Ethikrat 2011b, 149). Besides human patients, parents, children etc., there is an obligation to avoid suffering, pain or harm to animals and human-animal-mixtures (Deutscher Ethikrat 2011c, 47-51;55f.;109;et passim).

Existential Use of "Suffering": Who Suffers from What?

If we take a look at the findings talking about the suffering in an existential sense, we can ask who suffers from what and how to deal with this suffering. Obviously, the answer to the question "Who suffers?" entails the answer to the just raised question "Who is the object of the obligation to avoid suffering?" It is people with dementia and their relatives (Deutscher Ethikrat 2012b, 7f.;37), people with different sexual development (DSD) (Deutscher Ethikrat 2012a, 16;94;104f.;152f.;166;172;176), future children (Deutscher Ethikrat 2011b, 60;64;93;137;149), parents of disabled and ill children (Deutscher Ethikrat 2011b, 101;149), couples with an unfulfilled wish to have children (Deutscher Ethikrat 2011b, 113;144) and human-animal-mixtures (Deutscher Ethikrat 2011c, 67).

However, it is more interesting what they suffer from: Certainly, there are the diseases and disabilities these persons suffer from (e.g. dementia) – be it themselves having the disease or their relatives having it (Deutscher Ethikrat 2012b, 7f.). However, suffering is not only caused by disease, but even more by

social reactions to disease or, more in general, to being different; people with
dementia suffer from the loss of feeling secure and – similar to people with
DSD – they suffer from being socially excluded and being different (Deutscher
Ethikrat 2012b, 8; Deutscher Ethikrat 2012a, 16;152f). So, besides the physical
suffering, there is an ongoing emphasis on the emotional and mental suffering
which situations of illness, disease, disability or simply of being different may
cause. Some of this suffering is caused by persons – e.g. the suffering of people
with different sexual development who have been subjected to questionable
medical treatment. Other sufferings are caused primarily by society and its
way of dealing with the otherness of people. There is also suffering caused neither by a person nor by society but simply by a disease or genetic mutation no
one can be held responsible for.

How to Deal with Existential Suffering?

If we take a look at what the recommendations are on how to deal with these
sufferings, a first and interesting finding is that only rarely reference is made
to medical treatment. In normal situations, the avoidance or alleviation of suffering is certainly a crucial moral reason for medical treatment. But the ethical controversies discussed in the opinions seem in most cases to deal with
suffering which cannot simply be treated by medicine. Solely in the paper on
PGD, PGD is named as a way to avoid the suffering of a future child and of the
parents (Deutscher Ethikrat 2011b, 60;93;101;137). In regard to DSD, it has been
medical treatments which caused the suffering of persons with DSD, as those
treatments led to the disturbance of the persons' sexual identity (Deutscher
Ethikrat 2012a, 96;104f.;165f.). The way to deal with the suffering here is neither medical treatment nor simply alleviation, but societal acknowledgement
of the suffering caused to those persons (Deutscher Ethikrat 2012a, 105). For
people suffering from dementia, it is yet again not primarily medicine which
helps to alleviate pain, but the way the everyday practice is framed: continuity
of everyday practice is a way to alleviate the suffering caused by the ongoing
process of change (Deutscher Ethikrat 2012b, 54).

   Thus, alleviation of suffering is obviously an obligation in medicine, but the
ethical problems discussed by the opinions of the German Ethics Council are
about suffering which cannot be alleviated primarily by medicine.

The Principle of Care and Suffering

Taking into account that the moral principle of care is a "Trojan horse" by
which suffering becomes a topic of the ethical discussions in the opinions of

the German Ethics Council, it is worth taking a closer look at the aspects of this principle.

Damage, Harm and Suffering

The principle of care is interpreted as the principle of avoiding harm and of avoiding or alleviating suffering. The terms suffering, harm and damage (in German there is only "Leid" and "Schaden") do have different connotations but cannot be distinguished clearly. While "damage" ("Schaden") accentuates the objectivity, "suffering" ("Leiden") emphasizes the subjective aspect, and the english "harm" lies somewhere in between. Accordingly, someone can damage me and I will not suffer from it, even though I acknowledge the damage. To some persons, certain sorts of harm might even cause delight or lust, and in other cases people might just cope with certain harm and will not suffer from it, as a lot of aged people can cope perfectly well with otherwise objectively recognizable impairments and do not suffer from them, while others do suffer from the same impairments.

On the other hand, we can say the problem about suffering is that it causes harm. So, in everyday use, these different concepts overlap. They mark different areas in a semantic field of vulnerabilities, with the objectivity of damage on one end of the spectrum and the subjectivity of suffering on the other end. Yet none of these words is merely objective or merely subjective. The question may be asked, though, of whether the principle of care aims primarily at avoiding the rather objective damage done to someone or at avoiding the rather subjective suffering from this damage (or at least the possibility that someone may suffer from it).

Beauchamp and Childress interpret the principle of nonmaleficence as a principle to not "inflict evil or harm" (Beauchamp/Childress 2013, 152), which leaves room for both interpretations. The traditional ethical principle "primum nil nocere" and the legislative rule of Roman law "neminem laedere" both use concepts with a rather objective notion of damage (nocere and laedere). If we take the principle of nonmaleficence by word – according to its Latin roots – it simply means not to do any evil (non malum facere). This has two implications: (1) this moral principle is in its broadest sense about avoiding evil (malum); this includes damage, harm and suffering. (2) This principle is only about not doing evil to others and not about how to deal with evil others are otherwise confronted with. It basically says: "Do not be the cause of evil to others!"

Nonmaleficence and Beneficence

The moral obligation to alleviate suffering goes much further, because it does not only ask for who or what causes damage or suffering, but asks to prevent others from being harmed and to remove what causes harm to them. While not causing pain or suffering is one of the possible specifications of the principle of nonmaleficence (Ibid., 154), the duty to "prevent harm from occurring to others" and to "remove conditions that will cause harm to others" (Ibid., 201, 204) are specifications of the principle of beneficence. The obligation to alleviate suffering therefore falls under the moral principle of beneficence: recognizing someone is suffering implies to understand his or her wellbeing is impaired, and therefore there is a prima facie obligation to do him or her good, which in this case implies to alleviate their suffering. And yet again the question is: Does it make a difference to our moral obligation if we recognize damage, harm or suffering and if so, what is the difference?

The Normative Impact of the Suffering of Others

Concerning the opinions of the German Ethics council, there seems to be a tendency to use the German term "Schaden" ("damage" or "harm") as the more objective category, whereas the German term "Leiden" ("suffering") relies on a subjective response which presupposes at least a minimal consciousness. In due course, the concept of suffering is used only by reference to beings with at least minimal consciousness (including animals and human-animal-mixtures). This can, for example, be observed in the opinion on PGD, which refers to the *suffering* of the parents and the possible suffering of a possible future child suffering from a genetically caused disease (Deutscher Ethikrat 2011b, 60;64;93;101;137;149). The embryo, though, does not suffer, but has chromosomal or genetic *damages* (Deutscher Ethikrat 2011b, 7f.;13f.;31;141;143). Yet, it is precisely this damage that causes the suffering of the parents as well as the possible future suffering of the child this embryo might develop into.

This confronts us with a crucial problem concerning an ethically responsible use of "suffering": if the concept of suffering emphasizes the subjective response to damage, how far is it possible to ascribe suffering – and not only damage or harm – to other persons? The emphasis on the subjective dimension of suffering implies that the genuine form of speaking about suffering is the I-Perspective: "I suffer from … ". To ascribe suffering to someone else requires a reference to an at least intersubjective phenomenon. Thus, the question raised is: How do we know that someone else, who cannot express his/her subjective suffering – e.g. the future child in the case of PGD – will subjectively suffer from damage we might ascribe to him or her?

I would argue that there are certainly cases in which we can ascribe suffering to someone else. In cases, for example, of severe pain, we normally do not hesitate to conclude that the other person suffers – or would suffer from this pain if he or she would exist. This has to do with the human capacity for empathy, for which there is a sound empirical basis, as neuroscientific research has shown (Decety/Jackson 2004; Decety et al. 2017): the basic "building blocks" of empathy are "hardwired into our brain" (Decety/Jackson 2004, 71). Yet, the neurological reaction of a person observing pain in another person does not automatically lead to empathy and helping behavior. Decety & Cowell (Decety/Cowell 2014) have argued that empathy in itself is a highly complex system of precognitive neural reactions, affective perspective taking, emotional contagion and cognitive role taking. It therefore does not only consist of natural reactions to suffering, but also of cultural techniques by which the natural reaction to the suffering of another person is transformed into a prosocial, helping behavior that is triggered by the suffering of others. Fritz Breithaupt argues that empathy therefore requires a culture of empathy, especially narratives that enable a comprehensibility of the suffering we empathize with (Breithaupt 2017, 114-189).

If, for example, a couple concludes that a hereditary illness causing severe pain would result in the severe suffering of their child, everybody will very likely agree with this conclusion, because everybody takes severe pain as a comprehensible indicator of suffering. We know from our everyday experience that we are empathetic with someone suffering from pain. Yet there are a lot of other cases in which it might be less obvious that someone will suffer from harm; and therefore the question of how this ascription of suffering to another person really works, is crucial for an ethically responsible reference to the suffering of persons obliging us to a helping action. The crucial question seems to be: To what extent is it intersubjectively comprehensible or plausible that the other person really subjectively suffers from something? This is easy if there is an objective harm we all know we ourselves would suffer from – and we probably do know this because we can neurologically reproduce the suffering of the other person (without suffering ourselves). It becomes more difficult, though, the less the cause of suffering is intersubjectively reproducible. Asking for ethical criteria for this comprehensibility of suffering means to ask how our culture of empathy works.

I cannot solve this problem here; what I wanted to point out is the complexity of the moral principle of care and how it relates to the human phenomenon of suffering. The imperative "Do no harm" is not the same as "Avoid suffering" or "Alleviate suffering". Although the opinions of the Ethics Council seem to distinguish between damage/harm ("Schaden") and suffering ("Leid"), this difference is at the same time obscured by interpreting the principle of nonmaleficence as a principle of avoiding harm and alleviating suffering.

Considering the question of how the objective and the subjective aspects of damage, harm and suffering do relate to each other shows us why the question of how we recognize suffering in others and what impact this has on the moral status, is a crucial question not only for the ethics of animal rights. The question, to what extent we can ascribe suffering to someone else, is crucial for the ethical debates, for example, on PGD and Dementia Care. This is because it touches on the very foundations of morality by raising the question of what obligates us to help others who suffer, and what the limits of this obligation are.

Conclusions

In conclusion, first of all one has to recognize that, overall, the term "suffering" is rarely used in the opinions of the German Ethics Council. If used, it mainly refers to a subjective response to harm people suffer from. Rather, objective dimensions are described by other terms like damage, harm or impairment. "Suffering" enters the ethical debate by means of the moral principle of care, which is interpreted as the principle of avoiding and alleviating suffering. Therefore, the focus of the opinions is on suffering as something to be avoided or alleviated, and not on suffering as an irreducible part of human vulnerability.

The alleviation of suffering is certainly a crucial moral reason for medical treatment. By reference to the ethical concept of principlism it can be interpreted as a specification of the principle of beneficence. The principle of non-maleficence is about not causing harm or suffering. Most (but not all) of the discussed ethical problems in the opinions show, that there are other answers to suffering than medical treatment, because suffering often results not from illnesses, but from the way society reacts to someone being different because he or she is ill or impaired.

It remains a crucial ethical question, whether the obligation to avoid and to alleviate suffering aims at avoiding the rather objective aspect of harm, or at avoiding the rather subjective aspect of suffering from harm. This question certainly needs a much more intense discussion. I have only pointed out that this question is partly obscured in the opinions of the German Ethics Council. Dealing with this question requires a more detailed analysis of the concept of empathy, and of the moral obligations to help those suffering derived from this concept.

Bibliography

Act on the Establishment of the German Ethics Council (Ethics Council Act – EthRG), in: BGBl 2007, I, 31: S.1385. English translation online: https://www.ethikrat.org/en/the-german-ethics-council/#m-tab-0-ethicscouncilact (last access 04/10/2019).

Beauchamp, Tom L./Childress, James F. (2013): Principles of biomedical ethics, 7th ed., New York: Oxford Univ. Press.

Bentham, Jeremy (1876): An Introduction to the principles of morals and legislation, Oxford: Clarendon Press (reprint of the 1823 edition).

Breithaupt, Fritz (2017): Kulturen der Empathie, 5th ed., Frankfurt a.M.: Suhrkamp.

Decety, Jean/Cowell, Jason M. (2014) The complex relation between morality and empathy, in: Trends in Cognitive Sciences 18, 7: 337-339.

Decety, Jean/Jackson, Philipp L. (2004): The functional architecture of human empathy, in: Behavioral and Cognitive Neuroscience Reviews 3, 2: 71-100.

Decety, Jean/Meidenbauer, Kimberly L./Cowell, Jason M. (2017): The development of cognitive empathy and concern in preschool children: A behavioral neuroscience investigation, in: Developmental Science 2018, 21. Online: http://dx.doi.org/10.1111/desc.12570 (last access: 04/03/2019).

Deutscher Ethikrat (2009): Das Problem der anonymen Kindesabgabe (Anonymous relinquishment of infants: tackling the problem), Berlin: Deutscher Ethikrat.

Deutscher Ethikrat (2010): Humanbiobanken für die Forschung (Human biobanks for research), Berlin: Deutscher Ethikrat.

Deutscher Ethikrat (2011a): Nutzen und Kosten im Gesundheitswesen – Zur normativen Funktion ihrer Bewertung (Medical benefits and costs in healthcare: The normative role of their evaluation), Berlin: Deutscher Ethikrat.

Deutscher Ethikrat (2011b): Präimplantationsdiagnostik (Preimplantation genetic diagnosis), Berlin: Deutscher Ethikrat.

Deutscher Ethikrat (2011c): Mensch-Tier-Mischwesen in der Forschung (Human-animal mixtures in research), Berlin: Deutscher Ethikrat.

Deutscher Ethikrat (2012a): Intersexualität (Intersexuality), Berlin: Deutscher Ethikrat.

Deutscher Ethikrat (2012b): Demenz und Selbstbestimmung (Dementia and self-determination), Berlin: Deutscher Ethikrat.

Deutscher Ethikrat (2013): Die Zukunft der genetischen Diagnostik – von der Forschung in die klinische Anwendung (The future of genetic diagnosis – from research to clinical practice), Berlin: Deutscher Ethikrat.

Deutscher Ethikrat (2014a): Biosicherheit – Freiheit und Verantwortung in der Wissenschaft (Biosecurity – Freedom and Responsibility of Research), Berlin: Deutscher Ethikrat.

Deutscher Ethikrat (2014b): Inzestverbot (Incest Prohibition), Berlin: Deutscher Ethikrat.

Deutscher Ethikrat (2015): Hirntod und Entscheidung zur Organspende (Brain death and decisions regarding organ donation), Berlin: Deutscher Ethikrat.

Deutscher Ethikrat (2016a): Embroyspende, Embryoadoption und elterliche Verantwortung (Embryo Donation, Embryo Adoption and Parental Responsibility), Berlin: Deutscher Ethikrat.

Deutscher Ethikrat (2016b): Patientenwohl als ethischer Maßstab für das Krankenhaus (Patient Welfare as Ethical Standard for Hospitals), Berlin: Deutscher Ethikrat.

Liebsch, Burkhard (2014): Verletztes Leben. Studien zur Affirmation von Schmerz und Gewalt im gegenwärtigen Denken, Zug: Die Graue Edition.

Mackenzie, Catriona/Rogers, Wendy/Dodds, Susan (Eds.) (2014): Vulnerability. New essays in ethics and feminist philosophy, Oxford: Oxford University Press.

Schmidt, Jochen (2011): Klage. Überlegungen zur Linderung reflexiven Leidens, Tübingen: Mohr/Siebeck.

Tham, Joseph/Garcia, Alberto/Miranda, Gonzalo (Eds.) (2014): Religious Perspectives on Human Vulnerability, Dordrecht: Springer.

Suffering – an Increasingly Relevant, Though Ambivalent Concept in Bioethics

Claudia Bozzaro

Suffering: an Increasingly Relevant Concept in Bioethics

The notion of suffering is being used more and more frequently in bioethics and in medical and juridical practice, as evidenced by debates about controversial medical treatments at the beginning and the end of life (Green/Palpant 2014). Prenatal genetic testing, for example, is supposed to prevent so-called "needless" suffering (John Harris) (Majumder 2014, 404-430), while physician-assisted suicide or death on request are considered to be answers to "unbearable", "hopeless", or "intolerable" suffering (Duttge 2018; Sommerville 2014).

Interestingly, the notion of suffering is not only relevant as a rhetorical argument in bioethical debates, it is rather being applied increasingly in medical and in juridical practice. Intolerable or intractable suffering is, for example, a crucial medical indication used to legitimate palliative sedation at the end of life. Palliative sedation is an ethically controversial and currently more and more frequently applied therapy in palliative care. It is defined as the use of specific sedative medication to relieve intolerable suffering from refractory symptoms by a reduction of the patient's consciousness. Palliative sedation is considered as a treatment of ultima ratio, which means that it should only be applied in exceptional cases and only for terminally ill patients (Cherny et al. 2009).

Even in legal contexts regulating medical treatments, the notion of suffering is applied, for example, in the so-called right-to-die laws, which regulate physician-assisted-suicide and death on request in some countries like the Netherlands and Belgium (Belgium 2002; Netherlands 2002). In the Dutch legislation, unbearable suffering is one of the most important ethical and legal mandatory criteria applied to distinguish between legitimate and illegitimate wishes to die. In Germany, the BVerwG (Federal Administrative Court) stated in its decision dated March 2, 2017 set forth that people in an "extremely desperate situation" should have "the permission to obtain a lethal dose of pentobarbital sodium for the purpose of suicide" (German Federal Administrative Court (BVerwG), 020317U3C19.15.0, 2017). Here, suffering was the most important criterion the judges used to define an "extremely desperate situation" (Bozzaro 2018).

These examples show that the notion of suffering has a crucial normative role in bioethical debates and in borderline decision-making situations in medical and juridical practice (Callahan 2014). However, it is significant that this referring to suffering seems to have taken on such a high degree of plausibility and evidentiary nature that even defining the term itself seems to be superfluous. Indeed, the meaning of the term suffering and, more pecisely, unbearable or intractable suffering, is not defined either in the context of the practice of palliative sedation, nor in the legislations named above. This is insofar remarkable as the term does not serve merely as a mean of abstract orientation, particularly in these practical. Indeed, when the practical application of the term suffering is considered indepth, a number of problems arises that are connected to the term's vagueness and the normative value placed upon it in specific situations. In the following, I would like to present three concepts of suffering and their respective implications for practice as a first step. Afterwards, I advocate the need for a theoretical and ethical reflection and foundation of the concept of suffering as a basis for bioethics debates and for medical and juridical practice.

The Complex of Problems of Using the Concept of Suffering in Medical and Juridical Practice

The use of the term suffering in medical and juridical practice suggests that the definition of suffering is clear and well established. However, that does not reflect reality in any way as an accepted definition of the term does not exist (Dees 2010; Beijk 1998). Moreover, there is no agreement on the particular normative value of suffering as a basis for medical or legal decisions. This inconsistent understanding of suffering and its normative value raises several theoretical and also practice-relevant questions (Bozzaro/Schildmann 2018):

a) *The prerogative of interpretation* refers to the question: Who defines suffering in the particular contexts? On the one hand, suffering may be understood as a subjective experience. This would imply that only the suffering person, affected by the experience of suffering, can define if they are suffering. On the other hand, in order to use suffering as a normative criterion in intersubjective practice like in medicine or in law, a third-party (a physician or a judge) needs to assess the presence of suffering, as it is in their duty and (the medical and juridical) responsibility to decide whether, for example, palliative sedation is indicated or not, or whether a patient's wish to die is legitimate or not.

b) *Defining criteria for suffering* refers to the question: Which symptoms, conditions, and experiences should be taken into consideration to determine whether a person's suffering makes them eligible, i.e., for palliative sedation, or the right to die? The word suffering can be applied to different conditions and experiences ranging from symptoms, such as physical pain and dyspnea, to social conditions such as loneliness, or even existential experiences such as a sense of meaninglessness. So what do we mean by suffering when we refer to this concept in bioethical debates or in medical and juridical practice?

c) A third problem is centered on the *normative function of suffering*. If someone says, "I'm suffering," they are appealing for help. In this sense, the term has a strong normative function. In the context of palliative sedation or assisted dying, adjectives such as unbearable, intolerable, or intractable reinforce the normativity of suffering, as they express the urgency of intervention. In contrast, they also mark a difference between experiences that are bearable, tolerable, and tractable, and those that are not. But who decides when and which kind of suffering is bearable and which is not? Further: Are there limits to the duty to relieve suffering, or not?

Starting from the assumption that a significant number of answers to the controversial issues mentioned above hinge on our understanding of suffering, I will now shortly present three different accounts of suffering that I call respectively the subjective, the objective, and the social account.

Three Accounts of Suffering

The Subjective Account of Suffering

The "subjective account" was proposed by Eric Cassell, who developed a detailed concept of suffering as a merely subjective and all-encompassing experience in his widely received book *The Nature of Suffering and the Goals of Medicine* (Cassell 1991). The starting point of his reflections was a critique of the dualistic view of the human being in modern medicine. Due to this dualistic approach, modern medicine focuses on objective and measurable processes in the body and neglects the subjective experience of the suffering or ill person. Against this approach, Cassell claimed that suffering is experienced by persons and that persons are holistic entities. Accordingly, a person who suffers is always affected in all the dimensions that comprise their being (physical, psychological, social, existential, spiritual). Therefore, it is not valid to make a distinction between different types of suffering (e.g. between physical or existential suffering). Despite the fact that the source of suffering can be different – pain can cause suffering, as well as loss of dignity – suffering is always a threat to the integrity of the whole person. What is experienced as, and judged to be, suffering depends on individual interpretative patterns and values. Thus, "suffering is ultimately a personal matter – something whose presence and extent can only be known to the sufferer" (Cassell 1991, 35).

The Objective Account of Suffering

Stan van Hooft put forward a very different view of suffering in his paper *Suffering and the Goals of Medicine* (van Hooft 1998), published seven years after Cassell's book. Inspired by Aristotle's model of the soul, Van Hooft suggested four levels which compose the existence of human beings: 1. biological, 2. appetitive, 3. deliberative, and 4. contemplative. Each of these levels has, in his view of the human being, a *telos*, a goal, towards which it strives inherently. The fulfillment of the biological level is the basis of health. The fulfillment of the appetitive level is given when a human feels satisfied, at the deliberative level when they perform their tasks, and on the contemplative level from having a sense of meaningfulness in their life. Van Hooft claimed that, "suffering is to be understood as the frustration of the tendency towards fulfillment (telos) of these various aspects of our being" (ibid. 1998, 126). There are two crucial points in this concept that are different to Cassell's concept. Firstly, van Hooft asserted that suffering is not a function of consciousness. Therefore, suffering does not depend on the awareness and the judgment of the victim experiencing suffering: "Suffering is an objectively present condition of the person" (ibid. 1998, 127). Therefore, persons can be considered as sufferers even if they are not aware of their own suffering, as could be the case, for example, with newborns, coma patients, or persons suffering from dementia. In line with this assumption, suffering is accessible to third parties. Secondly, even if the four levels of human existence are interrelated and, therefore, a suffering experience occurring at one level can suffuse the whole being, this model allows the distinction and location of different types of suffering.

The Social Account of Suffering

Dutch philosopher Henri Wijsbek came to another understanding of suffering in his 2012 *article The Subjectivity of Suffering and the Normativity of Unbearableness* (Wijsbek 2012). He reached it by analyzing how the term suffering was being handled within the context of the practice of assisted dying in the Netherlands. According to Wijsbek's assessment, the presence of unbearable suffering is the most central of the six due care criteria set forth in the Dutch law regulating euthanasia. In the law itself, though, there is no definition of the term suffering. It is assumed, according to Wijsbek, that there are a number of situations that any person would see as being a state of unbearable suffering. In borderline situations, two institutions – the courts and the regional review committees – are responsible for working out a more exact contouring of the term.

a) When a case is handled by a court, the court decision serves further specification and restricts the meaning of unbearable suffering. For example, Dutch judges in the so-called Chabot Case (1994) established that psychic suffering also meets the criteria of unbearable suffering. In contrast, in the so-called Brongersma Case (2002), the court decided that being "tired of life" and feeling a sense of meaninglessness in old age are emotional states not allowed to be included in the criteria. However, currently there are new discussions about whether voluntary euthanasia should also be permitted for elderly people who are "healthy."

b) In addition to these juridical attempts to contour the term more specifically, there is a second institution that also has such linguistic normative power. Since 1999, five regional review committees have been promulgating their decisions about cases reported to them and reviewed by their members. These compile a collection of semi-juridical decisions which contain authoritative interpretations of the term in controversial cases. In 2005, for example, one of these regional review commitees accepted that anxiety of suffering in the future can be an aspect wgich makes current suffering unbearable.

In effect, as Wijsbek concluded, the criteria for unbearable suffering do not express what the patient considers to be suffering from which they can no longer bear. Rather, the term encompasses what Dutch society believes a patient does no longer have to bear. By this, the term says, "We, the Dutch political community, do not require you to bear this any longer" (ibid. 2012, 329). In fact, the unbearableness of someone's particular suffering is neither judged by the actual patient, nor – although indirectly – through the ascription by their physician. Instead, unbearableness is defined on the basis of a social norm in which all these aspects – the patient's subjective judgment, the ascription from their doctor – are compared with a view on the shared societal meaning of unbearable suffering. Thus, suffering is understood as a social norm and its more exact, contextual interpretation is ultimately defined by the majority within a society.

Implication for Practice

It becomes obvious, even based on the brief sketch of the three accounts above, that understanding suffering as a subjective, as an objective, or as a social concept has considerable implications for the application of the concept in medical or juridical practice. I will explore some of these implications in the following by sorting them into the three areas of controversies introduced earlier: a) the prerogative of interpretation of suffering; b) the criteria to define suffering; c) the normative function of suffering and of unbearable, intolerable, or intractable suffering for each of the three concepts.

a)   *Prerogative of Interpretation*

Cassell's subjective account clearly locates the control over assessment of suffering in the suffering person. Due to the fact that the experience of suffering has a subjective and personal nature, it further follows that there is hardly a reliable objective way to assess this state. For the medical and juridical practice, this implies that only the patient has the prerogative to determine if and when palliative sedation is medically indicated, or assistance in dying should be legitimate.

The obvious challenges associated with the acceptance of the subjective account of suffering are partially addressed by van Hooft's objective concept. In line with his view of distinct levels of functioning in a human being, it is possible to determine from a third-person perspective whether a person is suffering. Most notably and relevant for clinical and juridical practice, this concept allows an objective assessment of suffering according to intersubjective criteria. It follows, then, that control about the assessment of suffering, according to van Hooft, belongs to the healthcare or juridical professionals. This can even be the case when a person does not realize that they are in a state of suffering. Accordingly, such a concept would allow the use of palliative sedation for patients who suffer without realizing their state and/or without being able to communicate about this state, as it may be the case with patients close to death. Using this account of suffering, one could also argue in favor of assisted suicide or euthanasia for incapacitated patients who are not able to give their informed consent.

Wijsbek, in turn, assumes that in the context of an intersubjective practice, the interpretation prerogative finally has to be settled at the societal level. Suffering cannot be determined subjectively, and the assessment of an objectively present suffering by a third party is also insufficient. On the contrary, the definition of suffering is ultimately a result of a societal process of understanding and judgment.

b)   *Defining Criteria of Suffering*

Cassell's concept of suffering emphasizes not only the subjectivity of suffering, but also its holistic nature. In his view, the medical distinction often applied between somatic suffering (pain), on the one hand, and psychological/existential suffering, on the other hand, is no reasonable assumption. There is no further valid criterion for suffering apart from the subjective account of the affected person. Accordingly, Cassell supports the claim that psycho-existential or spiritual suffering should be considered as a basis for palliative sedation (Cassell/Rich 2010). The claim that, if assistance in dying is legitimate, then it should be legitimate for all types of suffering, would probably be regarded rather in line with this view.

In contrast, van Hooft's distinction between four levels of the human being would allow a more nuanced approach to the determination of suffering. It allows the location of suffering experiences at different levels and, thus, to differentiate between certain types of suffering. While van Hooft did not analyze decision making in palliative sedation or assisted suicide, in his work it seems much in line with his concept to distinguish criteria according to which palliative sedation or assistance in dying may be an option, or not.

Wijsbek pointed out that in practice, differences in experiences of suffering are being made apparent, whereby the limitation to physical experiences of pain in the context of assisted dying is increasingly being questioned.

c)   *The Normative Function of Unbearable Suffering*

As indicated, the normative and appellative character of the term suffering, and especially of unbearable, intolerable, or intractable suffering, has strong implications for clinical practice. It suggests that the person afflicted can no longer tolerate their situation and that they are immediately in need of help. However, depending on the understanding of suffering, the scope of medicine and law regarding suffering seems to differ. Following Cassell, medicine has an all-encompassing duty to relieve all types of suffering. If it was only the subject who can assess their own suffering, and if suffering was a holistic experience, it seems difficult to put limits to the use of palliative sedation or assisted suicide, once a person describes themselves as suffering.

This is different when we take van Hooft's position into account, which suggests that the duty of medicine/law to relieve suffering is limited only to those areas which can be addressed skillfully. According to van Hooft, this applies to both the biological and the appetitive level. From this point of view, palliative sedation would not fall within the scope of (palliative) medicine being an adequate answer to psycho-existential suffering. Instead, such use of palliative sedation could be criticized as a form of "medicalization".

Wijsbek, though, demonstrated that the normativity of suffering in Dutch practice is ultimately accorded through a societal consensus about what "is – or isn't supposed to be". With this, the term suffering no longer expresses the subjective perspective of the affected, meaning their values and ways of thinking about life, but rather a value judgment about life situations from the viewpoint of a society's majority.

Limits of Each Account

Each of these three concepts points to special problems.

Cassell put the prerogative of interpretation down to patients and placed few limits to the scope of (palliative) medicine and law regarding relief of suffering. Consequential, situations in which patients suffer – and especially when their suffering is unbearable or intolerable – exert considerable moral pressure on health care professionals and judges. Cassell's subjective and all-encompassing understanding of suffering provides no indication about where to draw limits regarding the duty of medicine to relieve suffering. In this sense, suffering cannot be used as a normative criterion to discern between cases where palliative sedation or assistance in dying is legitimate and where it is not.

On the other hand, a main limit of van Hooft's concepts is that a medical indication for palliative sedation or assistance in dying would only be accepted if one could demonstrate reliably and objectively that a patient is suffering. Given the pressure accompanying situations for patients whose suffering is caused by non-somatic sources, such a limit seems difficult to defend. In such a case, it may well be that a patient perceives suffering, but no action follows due to the limited ways in which suffering can be determined in an objective manner. Moreover, and relevant from a normative perspective, the objective approach to the assessment of suffering may, in practice, also be associated with a more paternalistic attitude to a patient, in the sense that doctors or others know best or better than their patients whether they are suffering or not. A similar problem arises with Wijsbek's concept. When it ultimately is society – through means of its court decisions – which maintains sovereignty over the definition of suffering and its normativity, this in effect curtails the autonomy of the individual, as their power to interpret their own condition has effectively been denied. Moreover, this practice leads to defining a number of conditions as "exceptions," and correspondingly, people who have these conditions are judged as being in situations of unbearable suffering. It is conceivable that people thus judged might feel unwanted by society, or even feel pressured to agree on certain treatments against their wishes.

Conclusion

Suffering is a normative indicative criterion of increasing significance in bioethics and in medical and juridical practice. The example of the three concepts of suffering demonstrates that suffering may be perceived very differently when it comes to a descriptive, conceptual view, and also in reference to its normative value. These differences at the theoretical level are in turn of central importance for the term's practical use because, as shown, very different practical implications and problems result from each of the three concepts of suffering.

According to my assessment, the current, dominant understanding of suffering in medical ethics, medicine, and law has been inspired – though usually in an implicit way – by Cassell, and above all places the subjective character of this experience is paramount. This can be explained by the fact that, among others, a subjective notion of suffering fits well into the trend of emphasizing and strengthening individual autonomy, which has occurred in the past decades. Further, this understanding of suffering reflects the manner in which 19th and 20th century philosophy considered this topic. In the 20th century, the subject matter of suffering was approached above all in the context of existentialism, phenomenology, and critical theory. Hence, those considerations no longer took place in a thinking tradition centered on the great system questions, as it was the case for example, in German Idealism. The focus of philosophical reflection was rather placed far more on the individual person with their existential and, especially, corporal experiences. Various authors have conducted analyses on individual experiences of suffering, such as pain, depression, and angst, etc. Thereby, they have provided us a valuable and indispensable basis for a better understanding of suffering.

However, this focus on subjective and individual suffering is problematic, especially when one wishes to apply suffering as a normative criterion within the framework of an intersubjective practice. This is because the understanding of suffering in a purely subjective manner ultimately leads to, as mentioned above, its normative function becoming obsolete, insofar as that does not allow an objective application, or a basis that can be communicated intersubjectively.

In this paper's introduction I pointed out that the normativity of suffering is expressed through its appellative character. This means that individual, subjective suffering is always a message to other people. Despite the fact that the suffering person may become lonely, or isolated, suffering itself has an intersubjective component. It points to an objective reality which all people who have access to the appellative character of suffering recognize as being "something that should not be". In my opinion, this objective, intersubjectively perceivable, and shapeable reality of suffering ought to be an object of intensified philosophical, social, cultural, and last but not least, theological reflection. This is because the practice of alleviation of suffering as applied in medicine and by law relies ultimately on a jointly shared understanding of suffering. By

this, though, I do not intent that the prerogative of interpreting what suffering
is should fall to a society's majority, as in Wijsbek's concept of social suffering.
Instead, interpreting and dealing with experiences of suffering in the framework of intersubjective interaction between the sufferer and their environment should be designed in order to bring the subjective and objective views
together. That also means that it possibly does not make sense to use the term
suffering in a strongly normative way. It may, indeed, be based on the difficulties described above and their correlations to respective suffering concepts,
that the term suffering can only be applied in a weak sense as a normative term
for orientation.

Bibliography

Beijk, M. M. (1998): Unbearable suffering: What is it, what causes it, and who deter-
mines it? In: Medisch Contact 53: 825-827.

Bozzaro, Claudia (2018): Urteil zur Erlaubnis zum Erwerb einer tödlichen Dosis
Natrium-Pentobarbital zur Selbsttötung: Eine Analyse aus ethischer Perspektive,
in: Deutsche Medizinische Wochenschrift 143, 10: 748-751.

Bozzaro, Claudia/Schildmann, Jan (2018): "Suffering" in palliative sedation. Conceptual
analysis and implications for decision-making in clinical practice, in: Journal
of pain and symptom management. Online: https://doi.org/10.1016/j.jpainsym-
man.2018.04.003 (last access 03/01/2019).

Callahan, Daniel (2014): Foreword, in: R. Green/N. Palpant (Eds.), Suffering and bioethics. Oxford: Oxford University Press, ix-xii.

Cassell, Eric J. (1991): The nature of suffering and the goals of medicine, Oxford: Oxford
University Press.

Cassell, Eric J./Rich, Ben A. (2010): Intractable end-of-life suffering and the ethics of
palliative sedation, in: Pain Medicine 11, 3: 435-438.

Cherny, Nathan I./Radbruch, Lukas/The Board of the European Association for
Palliative Care (2009): European Association for Palliative Care (EAPC) rec-
ommended framework for the use of sedation in palliative care, in: Palliative
Medicine 23, 7: 581-593.

Dees, Marianne K./Vernooij-Dassen, Myrra J./Dekkers, Wim J. et al. (2010): Unbearable
suffering of patients with a request for euthanasia or physician-assisted suicide. An
integrative review, in: Psycho-Oncology 19: 339-352.

Duttge, Gunnar (2018): Das "Leiden" als Passepartout im Recht? In: Bioethica Forum 11,
1: 30-33.

Green, Ronald M./Palpant, Nathan J. (2014) (Eds.): Suffering and bioethics, Oxford:
Oxford University Press.

Van Hooft, Stan (1998): Suffering and the goals of medicine, in: Medicine Health Care and Philosophy 1: 125-131.

Majumder, Mary A. (2014): Preimplantation genetic diagnosis and the prevention of suffering, in: R. Green/N. Palpant (Eds.), Suffering and bioethics, Oxford: Oxford University Press, 404-430.

The Dutch Termination of Life on Request and Assisted Suicide (Review Procedures) Act, 11/28/2000 (2002), in: Ethical Perspectives 9, 2-3: 176-81. Online: http://www.ethical-perspectives.be/viewpic.php?LAN=E&TABLE=EP&ID=58 (last access 05/03/2019).

Sommerville, Margaret (2014): Exploring the interactions between pain, suffering and the law, in: R. Green/N. Palpant (Eds.), Suffering and Bioethics. Oxford: Oxford University Press: 201-230.

Wijsbek, Henri (2012): The subjectivity of suffering and the normativity of unbearableness, in: S. Youngner/F. Kimsma (Eds.), Physician-assisted death in perspective. Cambridge: Cambridge University Press, 319-333.

German Federal Administrative Court (BVerwG), 020317U3C19.15.0, 03/02/2017, Online: https://www.bverwg.de/020317U3C19.15.0 (last access 03/06/2019).

The Belgian Act on Euthanasia of May, 28th 2002 (2002), in: Ethical Perspectives 9: 182-188. Online: http://www.ethical-perspectives.be/viewpic.php?TABLE=EP&ID=59 (last access 03/06/2019).

Suffering as Challenge for the Practice and Identity of Medicine

The Case of Body Integrity Identity Disorder

Tobias Eichinger

For some time now, a problem has been discussed in medical and medical-ethical literature that confronts physicians, psychologists, ethicists and social scientists with an unusual demand.[1] There are people who wish for the surgical removal of physiologically healthy and functional limbs. This phenomenon of desired amputation or voluntary mutilation is discussed among experts as *Body Integrity Identity Disorder* (BIID). Those affected experience a part of their body – usually an extremity – as not belonging to their own body, report a characteristic and serious alienation experience, according to which the affected part of their body is completely superfluous and disturbing for them. This feeling extends to the point that one's own physical integrity is experienced as fragmented, sensitively disturbed and incomplete, which in turn can have serious effects on identity formation and self-esteem. This condition, which can lead to considerable suffering, has often been lasting for many years, in many cases since childhood or adolescence. From the point of view of those affected, the only way to alleviate or heal their suffering is to remove the affected part of the body and thus to selectively damage themselves.

A central characteristic of BIID is the intense and persistent desire for a change of the existing body and the attainment of the desired body. The "overwhelming desire [...] to create a 'new' identity by fundamentally and irreparably damaging one's own body" (Pollmann 2007, 214), promises a new life free from suffering. Only in this way, they hope, is it possible for them "to achieve a complete body self" (Holzer/Stompe 2014, 38). For the same reason – to restore their physical integrity which is perceived as considerably disturbed – in some cases healthy people longingly wish for the elective separation of the spinal cord to bring about paraplegia, yet others feel the ardent desire to go blind. However, the majority of people affected by BIID would like to have their legs amputated (Stirn et al. 2010, 2). From a medical perspective, it is still unclear what the causes of this phenomenon are, and what an effective therapy might

---

1 This is a shortened and translated version of: Eichinger, Tobias (2015): Behandlungsziel Verstümmelung, in: G. Maio et al. (Eds.), Leid und Schmerz, Freiburg: Alber, 269-289.

look like.[2] What promises to be an effective and radical solution, however, is the actual fulfillment of the wish to remove the extremity, the elective amputation or the intended injury resulting in severe physical disability.

However, the compliance with amputation and mutilation wishes is an intervention that contradicts the traditional medical mission in a way that seems hardly more radical imaginable. *Primum nil nocere* has been the classical motto of medical art since antiquity. The fundamental and blatant discrepancy between BIID wishes and conventional medical orders and medicine's self-image is accordingly reflected in typical reactions and assessments that describe the phenomenon of the desire for amputation as "obscene" or "repulsive". Similarly unmistakable in his rejection, medical ethicist Arthur Caplan finds the concerns of BIID sufferers "absolutely nuts" and considers it "absolute, utter lunacy" to respond to such wishes for mutilation (Dotinga 2000). These statements seem to confirm the unquestionable incompatibility with responsible medical action from the outset, so that any further serious examination from a medical-ethical perspective would be unnecessary.

Extreme Wish-fulfilling Medicine

On closer inspection, however, it becomes clear that things here are somewhat more complex than the premature judgments that have been made, which are as striking as they are convincing, might suggest. First of all, an attempt must be made to examine, classify and understand the wishes of those affected. Clearly, amputation wishes are not wishes related to the treatment or healing of a disease or injury or the elimination of physical dysfunction. In this respect, they do not fall under the "therapeutic paradigm" (Eichinger 2013, 155) and can be understood as forms of wish-fulfilling medicine (Kettner 2012; Eichinger 2013). This term refers to the use of medical procedures and interventions that access the human body and mind to change them with the help of medication and operations, without any given illnesses or injuries. A paradigm has taken the side of the traditional concept, according to which medicine aims for and pursues the elimination of illness and suffering as humane act of help for people in need and distress, which rather addresses healthy people and understands medicine as a value-neutral "anthropo-technology" (Birnbacher 2012, 111). The range of services available to adapt the circumstances and conditions of one's own lifestyle to one's personal preferences, while making it more pleasant,

---

2 Discussions will include psychological, psychiatric, cognitive-behavioral-therapeutic as well as neurobiological explanatory models (Müller 2008; Stirn et al. 2010).

effective and successful, extends over the entire course of life, from measures of prenatal manipulation to the control and influencing of death and dying.

With options to adapt the psychophysical condition to individual preferences and ideals by medical means, the conditions achieved by the interventions in question can be assessed as better – 'better' according to generally shared understanding and comprehension of aspects. This applies for example if the goal is to be able to receive, process and memorize more information in a shorter time; or if the goal is to run faster, jump higher or stay awake and alert longer; or if one wants to have a more youthful and attractive body. However, this does not rule out the possibility that the goals pursued in detail can (and sometimes should) also be criticized, but these goals can first of all be characterized as improvements, since they concern an increase and intensification of skills and characteristics generally assessed as positive and desirable. With the help of wish-fulfilling medicine, their users hope and intend to become more beautiful, better, stronger, faster, younger, healthier, more alert, more efficient, more productive and more reproductive, better concentrated, more content and ultimately happier – all enhancements in this comparative sense aim at optimizing existing or achieving missing properties which are considered positive. It is not at all a trivial question whether a purely quantitative 'improvement' really is better, i.e. whether it is desirable in a comprehensive and profound, qualitative sense, and also in the long term. Nevertheless, most of the changes discussed in this way are changes whose attractiveness – at least for outside parties – is usually relatively easy to understand. In case of amputation and self-damage wishes, however, this is completely different. Not only the risks of implementation give cause for concern, but also it is above all the respective target itself that is highly disconcerting. Interventions, such as elective amputations and other forms of voluntary self-damage, do not only entail health risks and the risk of undesirable side effects – as a negative means to a positive end – due to the necessary procedural steps involved. But the goal in question itself, as is commonly believed, clearly constitutes damage, so that the intervention can be seen as a negative means to a negative end. Without the existence of a medical necessity, the body of a healthy person would be consciously impaired, harmed or injured by medical-technical means. In this respect, cases of self-requested damage are situated on the scale of change wishes directed at medicine to a certain extent opposite of positive (and hyperpositive) enhancement concerns.

At the same time, however, such wishes for 'groundless' injury, artificial disability and voluntary mutilation share with medical improvement wishes the difficulty of reconciling the treatments requested with the conventional medical ethos and the moral-professional integrity of medicine. As with measures to improve the physical or mental health of healthy people, there is no medical indication for claims of self-damage. However, not only ethically but also legally, this is the necessary condition for legitimate provision of medical services (Neitzke 2008, 53). Consequently, the sometimes odd concerns of self-damage can also be subsumed under the label of wish-fulfilling medicine, since medical knowledge and skills are to be used here exclusively based on an expressed wish, without medical necessity. However, in order to mark the empirically and ethically extraordinary nature of such measures, the term *extreme wish-fulfilling medicine* shall be used in this paper.

Body Modification to Design the Self

An important differentiating feature between the various forms of body modification such as the widespread procedures of tattooing, breast augmentation, nose modelling, or wrinkle removal on the one hand and the very rare cases of desired amputations and artificial paraplegia on the other hand, can be identified in motivation influencing factors. Interventions of wish-fulfilling medicine are essentially externally motivated and dependent on social factors such as status, communication and external impact. For example, cosmetic surgery clearly focuses on appearance and thus on physical characteristics that are and should be visible to others. Thus, the corresponding motifs are also essentially caused and shaped by the view from the outside. Already, reconstructive plastic surgery, the medical practice from which cosmetic-aesthetic surgery emerged, is based on this external motivation of social visibility. It almost inevitably deals with the external appearance and shape of deformed organs and tissue parts, aiming to restore them to the state before damage. A central motif here is the striving for normality. Visibly deformed and thus socially impaired people usually wish for nothing more than to look 'normal again'. Accordingly, the goal of plastic reconstructive medicine is to help the patient "to a 'normal' level of attention from others as far as possible" (Wiesing 2006, 144).

This form of normalization through medical action is diametrically opposed to the desired interventions at BIID. Here the (outwardly) normal and intact physical appearance is to be changed in order to achieve an obvious deviation from the norm of the healthy and functional body. While the hoped-for effect of something special and extraordinary consists in "increasing the attention of other people perceived as positive" (Ibid.), the opposite is true for amputation requests. BIID sufferers yearn for extreme body changes not because, but despite their social context. All case reports unanimously point out that people with BIID are well aware that their concerns by no means correspond to the culturally and medially conveyed body and beauty ideals of their environment, that the desired results are not evaluated by anyone else as an aesthetic benefit and that hardly any social advantages are to be expected from the operations. In this respect, the formation of identity through the fulfillment of amputation wishes is to be achieved by exactly the opposite of self-forming practices such as bodybuilding, breast augmentation, skin tightening or brain doping, which are all essentially aimed at socially conveyed and propagated values such as youthfulness, performance, beauty and – physical integrity.

Of course, as in the case of aesthetic medicine measures, amputation wishes also notoriously impose the question whether the implementation of the desired changes could affect the 'actual' cause of the suffering. What should be avoided at all costs, according to this, is "psychotherapy by scalpel" (Bayertz/Schmidt 2006, 55). This is particularly relevant because medical surgical operations carry out a form of self-design that not only proverbially gets under the skin, but which rather leads to results that cannot simply be discarded and changed again. Whether tissue is removed, injected, stretched, pierced, split, soaked with ink or artificially scarred – it's always about invasive and irreversible body manipulations that are desired and performed. Therefore, it is precisely the specific highlight of medical cosmetic changes of external appearance that one's own ideas remain durable and reliable. Thus, body modifications meet the needs of individual identity formation very well. Nowadays the body is more and more a medium of "identity management" (Holzer/Stompe 2014, 37).

Suffering from the Intact Body

Besides the blatantly non-conformist trait of the desire for self-damage, it is of great importance that the disturbed body image or the discrepancy between the ideal body image and the real body state, from which the affected persons suffer, has usually existed for a very long time, often for decades, without decreasing in intensity, or changing. What is remarkable here is that often very "precise notions regarding the 'line of demarcation' which separates accepted from unaccepted parts of the body [exist]" (Brugger 2011, 61) – amputation seekers can specify exactly where and how their nonintegrated forearm is to be cut off. In addition, many persons simulate the desired condition over long periods of time by bending their legs and moving around in public on crutches or in a wheelchair (Stirn et al. 2010, 2ff.). This simulation behavior called *pretending* is usually experienced as highly liberating and satisfying, which confirms, deepens and reinforces the already strong desire for amputation and self-damage (Kasten 2013). Short-lived and superficial preferences, which are to be implemented with the help of medicine, but which are always suspected to be of only limited duration and to appear and disappear as a result of fore-seeably changing fashions and trends, seem to be out of the question with amputation wishes. It is precisely the detailed and often repeated simulation of the desired disability that seems to meet important basic requirements for the fulfillment of serious medical interventions involving significant risks and resulting in hardly or irreversible body changes. At the same time, psychotic symptoms or bodily dysmorphic disorders can be excluded in the majority of cases (Stirn et al. 2010, 19).

The fact that people with a clear mind, full accountability and competence of judgement, knowledge of all alternative options and, above all, with many years of experience in pretending to be in the anticipated state of desire are well aware and constantly longing for the removal of an intact part of their body despite predominantly perplexed and rejecting reactions from other, shows that such desires for body modification are of existential significance for those affected. The fact that a serious, voluntary and deliberate impairment, such as the amputation of extremities, obviously runs counter to all common notions of functional efficiency, health and beauty, can be proof of the inten-sity and identification power of the desire. It also seems coherent and credible that those affected suffer to a considerable extent from the non-amputated condition and "see their functional capability as a person restricted precisely by the presence of the limb" (Brugger 2011, 62). Thus, for people with BIID the reversal of the usual notion of physical integrity can be observed. It is not the intact presence and unrestricted functioning of all body parts belong-ing to the typical physiological anatomical equipment of humans which is pre-supposed as a condition of a holistic feeling of integrity. Rather only through the absence of certain parts and thus the deviation from the usual scheme, the specific state of intactness, loyalty to the self, and authenticity as a person is attainable.[3] In this respect, desires for the separation of limbs for ultimate self-discovery correspond less to an understanding of the "body as a project" than to the opposing view that the physical body is "the last refuge of authenticity and ineluctable point of reference of identity" (Borkenhagen 2001, 55).

Yet, if wishes for medically unfounded mutilation exist and, in the sense of enlightened rationality, well-being and permanence, can be harmoniously integrated into the comprehensive ensemble of personal values, convictions and preferences of the person concerned – and at the same time the exis-tence of mental restriction, coercion or delusion can be excluded – it can be

---

3   Cf. on the different dimensions of the concept of integrity Arnd Pollmann (Pollmann 2007).

assumed that these are authentic wishes for specific forms of self-design.[4] The reported cases of BIID prove that, from the point of view of the person affected, authenticity or psychophysical integrity can carry more weight than physical (external) integrity. At the same time these cases can make the desire – initially appearing as "bizarre defect" (Brugger 2011) – visible as a 'real' desire of a suffering person that is to be taken seriously. If, moreover, a doctor refuses to professionally execute the desired impairment, automutilation, i.e. self-inflicting for its own sake remains a last resort; and since this form of 'self-help' generally carries considerably higher health risks than an intervention by technically experienced and authorized experts (Sorene et al. 2006), a serious assessment of the benefits and harms of this option must be carried out, especially from a medical-ethical point of view. Thus, in extreme exceptional cases a medically responsible action could mean the skillful implementation of the desired mutilation – as appropriate help for the reintegration of a diverging body-self-perception (Levy 2009).

This drastic consequence, which at first seems to question both the conviction of the respective physician as well as the ethical principles of medicine as a whole, however, lies not too far from the core mission of the centuries-old medical practice after all. One of the oldest and most fundamental tasks of medicine is to relieve pain and suffering where healing is not possible.[5] And it can be regarded as unequivocal that people with BIID suffer to a significant degree from the "subjective feeling of a bodily incompleteness in the face of a healthy physical body" (Kapfhammer 2012, 16).[6] As long as there are no convincing explanations of the causes, prevalence and classification of BIID, nor effective treatment options are known, the possibility of elective amputation cannot be excluded from the outset from an ethical point of view, given the suffering of those affected, which undoubtedly and actually exists. Otherwise, even in these extreme cases, there is the danger of patronizing the suffering person and falling back into paternalistic patterns (Schramme 2006, 165). That this may represent a great challenge for the foundations of the medical ethos is obvious, and is not to be downplayed either. A differentiated and unbiased

---

4 In addition, BIID sufferers are "usually intelligent, autonomous and successful people" (Stirn et al. 2010, 19). For the idea and requirements of a coherent wish clarification see Peter Stemmer (Stemmer 1998), on the identity forming dimension of wishes see Tobias Eichinger (Eichinger 2013, 63ff).

5 See for an antique example Hippocrates and for a more recent one the relevant formulation of the "goals of medicine" of the international Hastings Center project (Callahan et al. 1996).

6 Also see the first monograph published so far on the subject: "The suffering of those affected is immense because the wish cannot be implemented." (Stirn et al. 2010, 2).

examination and assessment of the handling of these few extreme cases nevertheless is required.

It might be suggested that the principle of non-maleficence could, under certain conditions, be subordinated to the objective of alleviating suffering, and therefore be restricted. Thus, it is possible that in individual cases personal psychophysical integrity is more important than physical integrity. It would be limiting and inaccurate to claim that people are ready to exchange their health for disability in fulfilling their desire for amputation. If one takes the tragic situation of BIID patients seriously, it must be stated that they rather demand to be able to exchange the suffering from their unfulfilled desire for the suffering from the resulting physical impairment (Kovacs 2009, 45). Accordingly, the fulfillment of an amputation wish would not only mean the transition from an externally intact body trapped in a (externally invisible) state of mental suffering to an externally handicapped body without corresponding mental suffering. There are many indications that carrying out the desired amputation could offer the possibility of finding oneself, and no longer suffering from a condition of "living as an amputee in a non-disabled body" (Craimer 2009, 55).

Relief from Suffering Instead of Disease Orientation

Phenomena of extreme medical wishes such as those of BIID patients show that clear definitions of "healthy" and "unhealthy" as well as of "normal" and "divergent" are no longer consistently practicable and acceptable. This does not mean that the concept of disease and the idea of health have completely lost their value as regulative ideals and points of orientation; nor that they will soon disappear altogether; the abandonment of the therapeutic paradigm as an orienting and standardizing framework for medicine as moral practice and profession with special responsibility and integrity would have alarming consequences (Eichinger 2013, 204ff). Though, in addition to the traditional disease orientation, new criteria and concepts are needed that are fit to take into account the reality of liberal societies and ideological pluralism. Here, various medical criteria and guidelines are conceivable – indispensable for this enterprise are goals and values such as freedom from suffering, integrity, authenticity, quality of life and well-being. That these variables can develop a normativity claim just as strong as the concept of disease has done for a long time is vividly illustrated by cases of BIID.[7]

---

7 The analogous example of the difficult classification of anorexia is also revealing here (Rebane 2012).

The fact that this shift in the fundamental values of medical practice, still in need of limitation and legitimization, does not have to result in a completely free and arbitrary *anything goes-policy* without control, is already evident in the mentioned candidates for contemporary criteria themselves. Aspects such as freedom from suffering, integrity and authenticity are far from being at the discretion of the individual. Medical activity would therefore not become the matter of uncritical and compliant fulfillment of contingent and idiosyncratic desires for free self-design and lifestyle according to personal taste. Precisely because the assessment of individual suffering can ultimately only be carried out by the person concerned, and precisely because the urgent necessity of medical services for the alleviation of suffering could be claimed all too quickly, a serious examination by an independent expert is more essential than ever.[8]

Medical judgement is therefore still required, if not to a greater and more complex extent than is the case with the objectivist paradigm of the restoration of health in functional terms. In order to adequately assess criteria such as integrity, authenticity and individual well-being, considerations are then also required that aim less at a functional normal state than rather vague and open concepts such as for example that of a good life. Narrative hermeneutic approaches promise to be a fruitful method for appropriate and differentiated acquisition of the individual history, the embedding and processing of disorders, and incisions within the psychophysical biography of the person concerned. When it comes to developing the meaning of an unusual desire for physical change (such as a desire for amputation), in order to find a successful solution, a narrative approach seems to be particularly promising (Slatman/ Widdershoven 2009). Thus, dimensions such as quality of life, happiness, identity, authenticity and other parameters come into view that were originally not necessarily and explicitly part of the specialist domain of the medical profession. Rather, the judgement and decision-making capacity of the individual concerned is stated as the determining competence. Ultimately, only the person who suffers, who is fundamentally disturbed in his integrity, who is severely impaired in his authentic self-discovery, can judge this. The interpretation sovereignty of the person in need of help regarding his or her condition, and (as far as possible) also regarding the ways of remedy, seems to be ethically undeniable. Here, ultimately, lies the decisive reason for the importance of avoiding paternalistic behavior towards suffering people drawn from traditional concepts of naturalness and normality – even if it may be counterintuitive in extreme cases and especially difficult for doctors.

---

8   A comparable difficulty arises notoriously with enhancement desires (Wehling 2011, 241).

Bibliography

Bayertz, Kurt/Schmidt, Kurt W. (2006): "Es ist ziemlich teuer, authentisch zu sein ... !" Von der ästhetischen Umgestaltung des menschlichen Körpers und der Integrität der menschlichen Natur, in: J.S. Ach/A. Pollmann (Eds.), no body is perfect. Baumaßnahmen am menschlichen Körper. Bielefeld: transcript, 43-62.

Birnbacher, Dieter (2012): Die ethische Ambivalenz des Enhancement, in: M. Quante/E. Rózsa (Eds.), Anthropologie und Technik. München: Fink, 111-125.

Borkenhagen, Ada (2001): Gemachte Körper: Die Inszenierung des modernen Selbst mit dem Skalpell, in: Psychologie und Gesellschaftskritik 25: 55-67.

Brugger, Peter (2011): Der Wunsch nach Amputation. Bizarre Macke oder neurologische Störung?, in: Ars Medici 2: 59-63.

Callahan, Daniel et al. (1996): The goals of medicine. Setting new priorities, in: Hastings Center Report 26 (Special Issue).

Craimer, Avi (2009): The relevance of identity in responding to BIID and the misuse of causal explanation, in: The American Journal of Bioethics 9: 53-55.

Dotinga, Randy (2000): Out on a limb, in: Salon.com, 08/29/2000. Online: http://www.salon.com/2000/08/29/amputation (last access 03/05/2019).

Eichinger, Tobias (2013): Jenseits der Therapie. Philosophie und Ethik wunscherfüllender Medizin, Bielefeld: transcript.

Holzer, David/Stompe, Thomas (2014): Körpermodifikation – (sub-)kulturelle und psychopathologische Aspekte, in: Spectrum Psychiatrie 2: 34-39.

Kapfhammer, Hans-Peter (2012): Fremdkörper im Leib, in: Psychopraxis 15: 15-17.

Kasten, Erich (2013): Body Integrity Identity Disorder – Körperidentität durch erwünschte Behinderung, in: Lege artis 3: 165-177.

Kettner, Matthias (2012): Enhancement als wunscherfüllende Medizin, in: A. Borkenhagen/E. Brähler (Eds.), Die Selbstverbesserung des Menschen. Gießen: Psychosozial-Verlag, 13-31.

Kovacs, Jozsef (2009): Whose identity is it anyway? In: The American Journal of Bioethics 9: 44-45.

Levy, Neil (2009): Autonomy is (largely) irrelevant, in: The American Journal of Bioethics 9: 50-51.

Müller, Sabine (2008): Body Integrity Identity Disorder (BIID) – Lassen sich Amputationen gesunder Gliedmaßen ethisch rechtfertigen? In: Ethik in der Medizin 20: 287-299.

Neitzke, Gerald (2008): Unterscheidung zwischen medizinischer und ärztlicher Indikation, in: R. Charbonnier et al. (Eds.), Medizinische Indikation und Patientenwille. Stuttgart: Schattauer, 53-66.

Pollmann, Arnd (2007): Ein Recht auf Unversehrtheit? Skizze einer Phänomenologie moralischer Integritätsverletzungen, in: S. an der Walt/C. Menke (Eds.), Die Unversehrtheit des Körpers. Frankfurt: Campus, 214-236.

Rebane, Gala (2012): Anorexia nervosa: psychische Störung oder Selbstoptimierung? in: A. Sieben et al. (Eds.), Menschen machen. Bielefeld: transcript, 211-233.

Schramme, Thomas (2006): Freiwillige Verstümmelung. Warum eigentlich nicht? In: J.S. Ach/A. Pollmann (Eds.), no body is perfect. Baumaßnahmen am menschlichen Körper. Bielefeld: transcript, 163-184.

Slatman, Jenny/Widdershoven, Guy (2009): Being whole after amputation, in: American Journal of Bioethics 9: 48-49.

Sorene, Elliot D. et al. (2006): Self-amputation of a healthy hand: A case of Body Integrity Identity Disorder, in: Journal of Hand Surgery 31: 593-595.

Stemmer, Peter (1998): Was es heißt, ein gutes Leben zu leben, in: H. Steinfath (Ed.), Was ist ein gutes Leben? Frankfurt: Suhrkamp, 47-72.

Stirn, Aglaja et al. (2010): Body Integrity Identity Disorder (BIID). Störungsbild, Diagnostik, Therapieansätze, Weinheim: Beltz.

Wehling, Peter (2011): Biopolitik in Zeiten des Enhancements. Von der Normalisierung zur Optimierung, in: S. Dickel et al. (Eds.), Herausforderung Biomedizin. Bielefeld: transcript, 233-250.

Wiesing, Urban (2006): Die ästhetische Chirurgie: Eine Skizze der ethischen Probleme, in: Zeitschrift für medizinische Ethik 52: 139-154.

Suffering in the Islamic Tradition and Its Meaning for Intercultural Medical Ethics

Tuba Erkoc Baydar, Ilhan Ilkilic

There have always been illnesses that become a source of sorrow, pain, and suffering for human beings, from ancient times until today. Cultural traditions have attempted to give these existential experiences a variety of meanings. In this process, interpretations often exceeded physically perceptible feelings. In this paper, we will describe and discuss the theological roots and meanings of the term suffering in the Islamic tradition. For this purpose, firstly the terms used in the literature in relation to suffering and their epistemological roots will be examined. Secondly, philosophical and Sufistic grounds for suffering found in the Islamic literature will be presented and their effect on the generation of juridical verdicts in Islamic ethics will be discussed. Lastly, the concept of suffering in medical ethics will be analyzed and its implications within an intercultural framework discussed.

In the second part of our article, we will discuss a real medical ethical case in an intercultural treatment situation, where the term suffering plays a central role. Our goal is to show which kind of suffering can be experienced by Muslim patients or relatives in concrete practice and how it can be discussed in an intercultural treatment situation. Studying the meaning of different terms of suffering in a value-pluralistic society is an interesting topic for further discussions and reflections.

Terms of Suffering in the Islamic Tradition

The most frequently used Arabic words in the Islamic tradition in relation to the suffering of human beings or the painful events they experience are: al-alam, al-musibah and al-bala. Among these words, the concept of "al-alam" in particular is a fundamental one used in moral philosophy that has an important place in the expression of philosophical considerations related to happiness (Kutluer 1995, 23). Therefore, this term will be discussed first; subsequently, a more comprehensive and superior concept, "al-musibah," will be examined. Finally, the term "al-bala," the expression most frequently used in the Holy Qur'an in relation to the suffering experienced by human beings, will be discussed.

© BRILL SCHÖNINGH, 2022 | DOI:10.30965/9783657715428_009

The lexical meaning of "al-alam" is "to feel pain" and it is used to express various perceptions such as pain, ache, twinge, etc. (Ibn Manzur 1997). In the Holy Qur'an and the hadith (sayings and teachings of Prophet Muhammad's), al-alam and the words derived from it are used in numerous places to denote both worldly and otherworldly suffering. Especially in many Qur'anic verses, the suffering that a human being will face in the afterlife due to his/her actions in this world is emphasized frequently (Qur'an 14/22).

The concept of al-musibah, on the other hand, is more comprehensive than that of al-alam. The word is derived from the root letters "s-w-b," whose lexical meaning is "suddenly pouring rain". In general, musibah is defined as "a situation faced unexpectedly and in spite of one's own will" (Ibn Manzur 1997). In the Holy Qur'an, it is stated that all musibahs that a person will face are written in a book (Qur'an 9/50-51) and they take place only with the permission of God (Qur'an 64/11). However, it is also emphasized that a person faces a musibah as a result of his/her own actions (Qur'an 26/30).

Another word term that is frequently used in the Islamic literature to express the pain and troubles that an individual bears is the term "al-bala". An examination of the lexical meaning of al-bala and its terminological usage reveals critical information about how troubles like illnesses are assessed in Islam; thus, of the three terms this one will be most closely elaborated up-on. The lexical meanings of this bala are suffering, sorrow, grief, trouble, discomfort (Ibn Man-zur 1997); and its usage as a term denotes serious troubles (al-Isfahani 2002). The word al-ibtila, on the other hand, shares the same root with al-bala but means "being tested." The meaning of the word ibtila points toward the connection between suffering and being tested. As a reflection of this connection, the Holy Qur'an describes the Prophet Abraham's attempt to sacrifice his son Ismail as "a tremendous bala" (Qur'an 37/107). There are also many other verses in the Holy Qur'an highlighting the connection between al-bala and al-ibtila. For exam-ple, the 155th verse of Surah al-Baqarah states: "And surely We will test you with something of the fear and the hunger and loss of wealth and lives and fruits, but give good news to the patient ones" (Qur'an 2/155). Also, in the 186th verse of Surah Al Imran God states: "You will certainly be tested in your wealth and yourselves" (Qur'an 3/186). In addition to these instances, it is emphasized in numerous verses (Qur'an 3/186) that suffering in this world due to illnesses, troubles, and sorrows is part of a test that all human beings are subjected to. That a person should regard all negative events happening in his/her life as a part of the test is emphasized not only in the Holy Qur'an, but also in various hadiths (Bukhârî "Riqaq" 28).

To summarize, the meanings of the words al-alam, al-musibah and al-bala in the Islamic lit-erature and the ways they are used in the Holy Qur'an and the hadith of the Prophet Muhammed reveal that all the suffering that human beings experience in this world requires profound interpretation. Considering that suffering is meant to educate people, help them mature, and give them the strength and will to tolerate and endure in the face of the heavy troubles of this life, one of the most important concepts related to suffering is the concept of being tested, as has been accepted by Islamic scholars in general. Their opinions on this subject are presented below.

Comments on Suffering by Muslim Scholars

The first Muslim philosopher, al-Kindî (d. 866), connoted that suffering, including the suffering that comes from an illness or suffering that results in death, is an inevitable aspect of life, and that if an individual does not suffer a little in this world, it means s/he does not exist at all (Kutluer 1995, 23). Al-Kindi, in his treatise on suffering, states that living in a universe that is subject to the law of being in constant formation and deformation makes it natural that human beings should suffer (ibid.). According to him, what should be done in this case is to endure and transcend these sufferings and prepare for the afterlife, in which there is no pain. His student, Abu Zayd al-Balkhî (d. 934), followed his teacher in this advice, asserting that there is no means to end physical and spiritual suffering in this world entirely, despite all the resources for treatment provided by medicine and the moral sciences; freedom from suffering can happen only in Paradise (ibid.). Two other prominent philosophers of the Islamic world, al-Razî (d. 925) and Ibn Miskawayh (d. 1030) also wrote treatises on the issue of suffering, endorsing approaches similar to that of al-Kindî.

This approach developed by the Muslim philosophers, which holds that the suffering of this world will end in the afterlife, being part of the test that all human beings are subjected to, is also emphasized by other Muslim scholars. For example, one prominent Qur'anic commentator, al-Zamakhsharî (d. 1144), clearly indicates that a musibah is given to a person in order to test him/her (al-Zamakhsharî 1947, vol. 2, 232-233). Theologians also opine that musibahs such as illnesses faced by human beings are a means of education, testing, and warning both for those who suffer them and those around them (al-Mâturîdî 2003, 351-485). Similarly, Sufis (a Sufi is a member of an Islamic Mystical School) also see al-bala and al-musibah as means of being tested (Sarraj 1996, 345). For example, according to Sarraj al-Tusî (d. 988), there are three kinds of test that occur through al-bala and al-musibah: they can be a means of punishment for sins, a means of purification and redemption, or a means of spiritual elevation (Sarraj 1996, 362). It is important here to note that the Sufis interpret the suffering of human beings in this world in three positive ways. Spiritual elevation is the one that attracts special attention: According to Sufis, suffering due to illnesses or other sources of trouble is a means to reach spiritual positions that one cannot reach under normal circumstances.

As Sarraj al-Tusî emphasizes, one of the most important reasons to be patient in the face of an illness, musibah, bala, or suffering is that it is heralded that there will be a reward for those who endure and are patient. Indeed, it is stated in Qur'anic verses (Qur'an 2/86) that suffering, pain, troubles, problems, and the distasteful things of this world should be regarded as means of being tested, and those who are patient will be rewarded in the afterlife. In this context, the Prophet Muhammed answered a question about the plague, which He described as a suffering given by God to any one of His servants whom He wishes well, and that it is a blessing for those who believe and those who bear it patiently, hoping that God will reward them like a martyr (al-Tirmidhi "Zuhd" 57). Similarly, it is mentioned in many hadiths that all exhaustion, illnesses, grief, pain, anxiety, and any kind of trouble, including even a prick, is penance for the sins of Muslims (al-Bukharî "Merdâ" 3). Following these verses and hadiths, Islamic scholars have reached a consensus that suffering in this world is a means to be forgiven for the sins committed in this world (al-Alusî n.d.,vol. 5, 152). For example, Imam al-Mâturîdî (d. 944) stated that those who are tested will find mercy in the end (al-Mâturîdî 2003, vol. 2, 505), and most scholars stated that those who are suffering in this world will be rewarded in the afterlife (al-Juwaynî 1992, 247; al-Ghazâlî 2008, vol. 1, 287; al-Râzî 1986, vol. 1, 350).

Suffering in this world has other meanings and purposes besides redemption, including to bring a beloved humankind closer to God, to remind a servant of the reason s/he was sent to the earth, to erase a servant's sins, or to promote a servant's place in God's regard. In addition, suffering, illnesses, and troubles can be consequences of the injustices and wrongdoings committed by people. In this context, the reasons for the suffering of babies who committed no sin, children who cannot distinguish between right and wrong, or people who are not of sound mind, should be examined. The reasons for the suffering of these people have been examined in the theological literature under rubrics such as al-alam and al-ivaz. It is clearly stated that children who are not old enough to be held responsible are not subjected to problems and alam because of someone else's sins (e.g. their parents'). The suffering of children, mentally ill people, etc., can be both a means of promoting the spiritual position they will hold in the after-life and a means of testing those who are around them to see how they will treat them. In this context, the Mutazilî scholar Qadî Abd al-Jabbar (d. 1025) said "a child is sinless, so s/he cannot be punished" and thus pointed out that the suffering of children cannot be seen as punishment (Qadî Abd al-Jabbar 2013, vol. 2, 286).

As discussed above, suffering and troubles are a means of testing various virtues of human beings like patience, sincerity, faith, and commitment to God. As seen in the parable of Job (Qur'an 21/83, 38/42), it is meant to raise an awareness that pain and suffering given by God are given due to an underlying wise reason, and the best thing is to be patient instead of rebelling against Him. Therefore, according to Islam, seeing illnesses faced in this world as purely negative phenomena is a misevaluation of the issue. Gains and losses should be evaluated taking the afterlife into consideration. The reason that the concepts of beneficence and evil are referred to frequently in the Holy Qur'an and the Sunnah (i.e. the tradition of the Prophet Muhammad) is that an individualistic determination of benefits and losses does not correspond to the fundamental demands of religion (Aybakan 2002, 131). The Qur'an also reminds its reader that something should not be regarded as good or bad just by looking at its superficial outcomes (Qur'an 2/216). A very rich and deep debate has been going on regarding the nature of good and evil within Islamic thought (al-Taftâzânî 1998, vol 1, 375-419). As al-Ghazalî (d. 1111) suggested, it is important to keep in mind that evaluations such as good and evil or benefit and loss are necessarily relative, for there is no objective measure for these concepts (al-Ghazâlî 1994, vol 1, 56-57). Another important question that should be kept in mind is whether something that is good specifically for the body is or is not also good for somebody in general. Acknowledging the transcendental aspect of the human being necessitates a negative answer to this question.

The Meaning of Suffering at the End of Life

The idea that a life in pain is not worth living, as claimed in debates regarding issues like suicide, ending life, and euthanasia, is not an acceptable position in Islamic thought. Indeed, Islamic anthropology treasures human life, which it sees as being sacred above everything else, under all circumstances. The idea that a person in the terminal stage of life, in a vegetative state, or in intensive care is not a person but only a living organism cannot be defend with the normative terms of Islamic ethics. Just as it is forbidden to kill oneself due to pain, killing someone else is not approved in Islam, either (Baydar 2017). For example, prominent Islamic scholar al-Ghazalî discussed elaborately whether or not it is permissible to kill someone in unbearable pain, In his book al-Waseet, al-Ghazalî eventually gave a negative answer to this question, saying that even if it is known that the person in pain is going to die in a short period of time, no one has such a right and it is not permissible to kill him/her (al-Ghazalî 1997, 522). As can be seen in al-Ghazali's statement, the fact that a person is in grave pain and the absence of hope to treat him/her are not valid reasons in Islamic jurisprudence to legalize taking his/her life, the reason being that Islamic jurists accept the legal right of security of life even for people who are suffering from a terminal disease (Arabic marad al-mawt), because having a terminal disease does not change the fact that killing him/her is classified as a deliberate murder.

In the modern age, Muslim scholars take different approaches to the topic of terminating or deciding not to initiate treatment (Rashvan n.d., 791) The first approach, which holds that treatment should be continued unconditionally, argues for the necessity of treatment before death even in hopeless cases (see Ilkilic 2006, Ilkilic 2014). Proponents of this approach see no distinction between active and passive euthanasia because the purpose in each case is the same; thus they hold that passive euthanasia, like active euthanasia, should be impermissible. Another approach, while not claiming that treatment before death is obligatory, still considers it to be recommended (Rashvan n.d., 793-94).

On the topic of treatment being terminated or rejected, Qaradawi – an Egyptian Muslim theologian – views treatment as obligatory in cases where there is hope of a cure, but also views it as neither obligatory nor encouraged for cases where experts agree that it will have no effect toward curing the patient and will only prolong the illness. Moreover, Qaradawi holds that these cases should not be thought of as falling within the scope of the euthanasia debate (Qaradawi 2016). Abdulaziz Sachedina – a Muslim Scholar living in the USA – argues that because active euthanasia is based in a "right to die", it is not acceptable from an Islamic perspective. Passive euthanasia, on the other hand, means "allow to die", and in that perspective, it is unnecessary for treatment to be applied to terminal patients with the aim of their survival (Sachedina 2009).

Suffering in an Intercultural Medical Ethical Case

Following on from the above analysis of the term suffering in the Islamic tradition, we will now discuss a real medical ethical case in an intercultural setting and reflect on the problems of different ethical dimensions of suffering.

Case

A six-day-old child of Turkish Muslim parents is suffering from type II oto-palato-digital syndrome (OPD), a rare genetic disease leading to severe anomalies in the formation of several organs. Previously, the mother had lost another child in the 37th week of gestation. In a second pregnancy, she had suffered a miscarriage in the 17th week. In this case, the fetus was examined and a molecular genetic test found the presence of a type II oto-palato-digital syndrome (OPD-II syndrome). On that occasion, the mother was diagnosed as a carrier of the relevant X chromosomal mutation. The case described here regards her third pregnancy. During the fourth month of gestation, the parents presented at a specialized clinic where the OPD-II syndrome was diagnosed in the fetus, too. However, the parents decided to leave the pregnancy to its natural course and did not seek any further consultation or care.

OPD-II syndrome is extremely rare and leads to a wide variety of symptoms. In most cases, the decisive factor for the course of the disease and the prognosis is the degree of pulmonary hypoplasia. The child in this case suffered from respiratory insufficiency at birth, due to which it needed to be intubated for artificial respiration. In addition, clinical and laboratory data indicated renal failure in the newborn. In principle, it was conceivable to step up ventilation and to apply renal replacement therapy. Increase in ventilation would only have delayed an inevitable respiratory failure. Renal replacement would have had to continue life-long, as it could not be expected that the child would receive a donor organ, considering its severe primary disease.

Without intensive mechanical support, the child was not viable; even with the use of machines – esp. the ventilator –, most likely the child would have been kept alive only for a very short time span.

With the help of a relative of the parents serving as an interpreter, a consultation was undertaken. In order to not prolong the suffering, the German medical team suggested refraining from providing maximal therapy and limiting the extent of therapy. However, the parents requested a continuation of all life-prolonging measures for their child, even if there was no prospective of cure. They emphasized that their decision was based on their Islamic faith. Had they decided otherwise, they would not be able to justify their action in front of God in the Other World.

Different Meanings of the Term Suffering

In this case, we find a conflict in the decision-making between the parents of the sick child and the healthcare team regarding the determination of the therapy goal. Due to the child's futile situation, the team argues that the current therapy should not be extended through other interventions, even if this attitude caused the early death of the patient. Additional medical intervention would not only delay the expected death of the child but also prolong the child's suffering. In order to not extend the child's suffering, medical interventions should be limited to preventing hunger, thirst, fear, and pain.

The parents argued against this position. In their opinion, all available interventions needed to be applied in order to lengthen the life of their child. These interventions would have to be applied even if they only delayed the child's time of death. Even a survival of the child for only a few days or hours would be valuable and desirable for the parents. Their arguments for this position and their request are essentially characterized by religious beliefs. In their view, according to the Islamic believe people are obliged to save human life and to deploy all existing tools for lifesaving even in futile situations. Therefore, the parents could not accept any other decisions because they were unable to take the responsibility on Judgment Day in front of God. If they accepted the suggestion of the medical team, this would cause a great suffering for them in their afterlife.

In this conflict, we find various concepts of suffering with different characteristics. The notion of suffering held by the medical team arises in the context of the natural sciences and it is more objectively based in physical perceptions. This kind of suffering can be described as being verifiable through medical tests, if necessary. But the term suffering as used by the parents has a different ontological character and belongs more to the afterlife. Consequently, they associated other situations and spiritual consequences with this term. For the parents, accepting the decision of the medical team constituted a suffering in itself. For them, prolonging life in a futile situation through intensive medical care is not the suffering, but rather the situation arising from the limitation or withholding of intensive care and consequently the death of the child is what they see as suffering.

At first, we should be aware of the different meanings of the term suffering, which is shaped by cultural values and norms, in order to reach an ethically justifiable consensus. Secondly, we should try to answer the following questions:
– How should these different terms of suffering be communicated successfully?
– What is the ethical meaning of the coexistence of different terms of suffering?
– Which other normative terms, apart from suffering, are problematic in this case?

The Child's Best Interest in an Intercultural Setting

Presumably, the parties to the conflict exchange information about their different understandings of suffering and they realize that there is a disagreement. Nevertheless, they need to take further steps to reach an ethically justifiable consensus. Only being aware and having information about these different meanings of suffering is not enough to find a solution. In this context, we need a central ethical norm that can help us to assess different options for action. In such cases, the child's best interest as an ethical norm needs to be considered. This normative term may help us think about concrete decisions and interventions and also evaluate these actions.

Although ethicists and lawyers all around the world have come to a general consensus regarding the significance of the child's best interest, there is still controversy among experts concerning the criteria and definition of this ethical norm (Fleischmann 2016; Stuhlinger 2005, 153-165). For example, experts have criticized the absolute prioritization of medical facts as the deciding criterion concerning the child's best interest (Dörries 2003, 116-130; Glannon 2005). The focus on medical parameters permits objective criteria, but at the same time, it is also defective in that it omits important facts that equally pertain to the child's well-being. It is rightly argued that psychological, emotional, social, and cultural needs and their implementation need to be taken into consideration in the decision-making process (Dörries 2003, 124).

Even if, from an ethical perspective, there are good reasons for supporting the consideration of comprehensive criteria that include cultural values, it is important to keep in mind that this broadening will bring subjective evaluations and decisions with it. On the one hand, the child's best interest will benefit from the application of such a comprehensive catalog. On the other hand, it will cause the choice of criteria to become more subjective and allow more scope for varying interpretations. Thus, it will become increasingly more complex and difficult to find a solution among conflicting parties. It will then become necessary to agree a hierarchy and reach a consensus concerning prioritization in order to ensure the adequate application of these criteria. However, in a pluralistic society it will not be possible to establish this procedure without conflict. In those cases questions like "how does one act if the consideration of cultural values conflicts with the medical criteria of a pluralistic society" may arise (British Medical Association 2001).

Opportunities and Challenges in an Intercultural Ethics Consultation

In our case, we see how parents and the healthcare team ascribe different normative meanings to the terms involved. For the parents, the avoidance of the child's suffering does not have the same moral importance as it has for the healthcare team. The challenge to communicate these differences respectfully is demanding for both sides. Moreover, the normative term "child's best interest" is not easy to define for concrete actions. Additionally, language and cultural barriers in the communication between the child's parents and the medical team exist because the child's parents, with Turkish background, are not able to speak German very well. An ethics consultation could help in this complex case. Within the scope of this consultation, what is needed is a professional culturally sensitive moderation of the communication between the conflict partners. Additionally, a professional interpreter is needed to perform not only a simple interpretation, but at the same time needs to be able to convey the accurate meaning of central terms, which is a really daunting task.

Therefore, as has been argued in the literature, in such cases the interpreter should be not only bilingual but also bicultural (Snell-Hornby 2007, 86-94).

With the implementation of an appropriate communication, the ethics consultation should try to find common ground between the parents' wishes, the course of action preferred by the physicians, and Islamic norms and values. As discussed above, the scientifically describable suffering is common to the Islamic tradition. We found that suffering in the context of medicine could be interpreted in several ways. In the current Islamic medical ethics discourse, some Muslim scholars understand suffering at the end of life in terms similar to those of the medical team. According to them, if there is no possibility of healing or improving the quality of life, medical treatment can be limited or discontinued. For them, if the limitation of therapy leads to the death of the patient in a medically futile, this situation cannot be judged as killing the patient but letting him/her die. To inform the parents about this position and argumentation could give the parents a different perspective and may help us to reach a consensus. If we are to explain these specific arguments and existing theological positions, we need an ethics counselor with intercultural competence (Ilkilic 2017, 24-30). If this person does not have special information about Islamic medical ethics, he/she can invite a Muslim Theologian with special competence in medical ethical issues.

At the second stage in the process of communication, the parents can be confronted with the following – doubtless emotionally taxing – question: "What would you wish for yourself if you were in the place of your child?" This question – in spite of some problems it involves – should give the parents an opportunity to take a distance from their initial position and to change and reflect their decision and attitude.

Concluding Remarks on the Case

In summary, it can be argued that as an adequate approach to this kind of conflict, we have to consider the role and the ethical significance of normative terms like "suffering" and "the patient's best interest". Because professional, cultural and religious values essentially shape decisions and attitudes of the conflict partners, they must also be considered in an ethics consultation. Therefore, in this case, where parents request maximal therapy in a medically futile situation, it is important to make decisions accessible to the conflicting parties not only via their underlying arguments, but including cultural and religious foundations of the respective attitudes. Hence, an intersubjective objectifiability of one's own value system is required. What is needed is not merely a linguistically adequate communication, but in addition we have to gain access to the cultural worldview and the conception of the human being it is based on.

The underlying analysis has pointed out that suffering, medical futility, and the ethically appropriate course of action following from them, especially in intercultural therapy settings, cannot be reduced to a single scientific criterion. We have seen that taking cultural aspects into account and integrating them in an ethically adequate way into the decision-making processes in medically futile situations raises a number of difficult questions. An ethically adequate approach to conflicts arising at the end of life requires not only a response to these questions, but also a balance between conflicting values and different meanings of normative terms needs to be found. This balancing act opens up another range of issues, due to the confrontation of culturally-based differences in the attribution of values. Such diverse attributions of values to conflicting normative terms have not yet been sufficiently taken into account in the international medical ethical debate. Looking back, we can see that we are in need of elaborating concepts for dealing with this kind of divergent value attributions. In a value-pluralistic society, those endeavors need to embrace different culturally based value systems.

Conclusions

Every cultural tradition has its own term for suffering, shaped by the history of that tradition. Not only personal experiences in one's own social environment, but also culturally-shaped normative terms influence the value system of a person. If we consider that such value systems are decisive for many decisions and attitudes, then the importance of normative terms especially for medical ethical decisions at the end of life will become clear, as such situations are existential borderline experiences, where the understanding of the self with regard to normative terms gains exceptional meaning.

Above, we have discussed the theological roots and several intellectual dimensions of the term suffering in the Islamic tradition. In sum, we may emphasize that the Islamic tradition promotes accepting suffering, which is regarded as an essential part of the life in this world, and coping with it by attributing meaning to it, instead of denying, dismissing, or temporarily forgetting it. The suffering of this world will have an effect on the afterlife, as it is a means of being tested in this world. Furthermore, in the Islamic tradition, pain and troubles are considered to have a role in training people, helping them to mature, and giving them the strength and will to tolerate and endure in the face of heavy troubles of this life. In spite of these positive spiritual interpretations, it is not right to conclude that suffering is a desirable and ideal situation according to an Islamic image of humankind.

In the second part of our article, we looked at the practical consequences of this term in a concrete medical ethical case that had arisen in an intercultural treatment situation. In this case, we find different understandings of the term suffering, raising complex and challenging ethical issues. Firstly, we would like to emphasize that if modern medicine wants to treat people from several cultures with an egalitarian claim, medical practice should be opened to normative terms like suffering from the perspectives of different cultural traditions. The main difficulty seems to be how these terms can be implemented in concrete cases. Given that such issues are topics of the social sciences, they should seek and find appropriate answers. Secondly, we argue that classical traditions like the Islamic tradition should concretize their own normative terms for the problems of modern times, especially of modern medicine. Even if there are a lot of studies and discussions in the Islamic world about the ethical issues of modern medicine, we think that we need more specific research on these issues with regard to the complexity of the ethical problems in modern medicine.

Bibliography

al-Âlûsî, Shihabuddin Mahamud b. 'Abd Allah al-Alusi, al-Baghdadî (n.d.): Ruh al-Ma'anı fi Tafsir al-Qur'an, Beirut: Dâr al-Ihya at-Turâs al-Arabî.

al-Bukharî, Abû 'Abd Allâh Muḥammad ibn Ismâ'îl Ibn Ibrâhîm ibn al-Mughîrah Ibn Bardizbah al-Ju'fî (n.d.): Sahih al-Bukhârî, Istanbul: al-Maktabat al-Islamiyye.

al-Ghazâlî, Abu Hamid Muhammad b. Muhammad (1994): al-Mustasfâ min Ilm al-Usûl, Beirut: Dar-al Arqam.

al-Ghazâlî, Abu Hamid Muhammad b. Muhammad (2008): Ihya al-Ulum al-Din, Cario: al-Maktaba al-Tavfekiyye.

al-Jassas, Abu Bakr Ahmad b. 'Ali al-Razi (1996): Ahkâm al-Qur'an, Beirut: Dar al-Kutub al-'Ilmiyya.

al-Juwaynî, Imam al-Haramayn (1992): Kitâb al-Irshâd, ed. Esad Temim, Beirut: Müessese al-Kutub as-Sakâfiyya.

al-Maturidî, Abu Mansur (2009): Tawilât al-Qur'ân, ed. Muhammad Masum Vanlıoğlu, Istanbul: Mizan Yayınevi.

al-Maturidî, Abu Mansur Muhammad b. Muhammad (2003): Kitâb al-Tawhîd, ed. Muhammed Aruçi, Ankara: T.D.V. puplication.

al-Qâsânî, Abû Bakr (1997): Badâi' al-Sanai' fî Tartîb al-Sharai, Beirut: Dâr al-Kutub al-Ilmiyye.

al-Qashanî, Abd al-Razzaq (1966): Sharh al-Fusus al-Hikam, Egypt: Mustafa al-Bab al-Halebî.

al-Razî, Muhammad b. Umar (1986): al-Erba'în fî usûl al-dîn, thk. Ahmad Hicazi al-Sekka, Cairo: Maktabah al-Kulliyât al-Azhariyyah.

al-Sarakhsî, Muhammad b. Ahmad b. Abi Sahl Abu Bakr (1982): al-Mabsût, Istanbul: Çağrı Publications.

al-Taftâzânî, Sa'ad al-Din Masud Ibn Omar Ibn Abd Allah (1998): at-Talvîh ilâ Kashfi Haqâiq al-Tanqih, thk. Muhammed Adnan, Beirut: Dâr al-Erkam b. Abu al-Erkam.

al-Zamakhsharî, Abu al-Qasım Jarallah Mahmud b. Omar b. Mohammed (1947): al-Kashshaf 'an Haqa'iq al-Tanzil, Beirut: Dâru'l-Marife.

Aybakan, Bilal (2002): "Zarar", TDV İslam Ansiklopedisi (Encyclopedia of Islam), Ankara: Türkiye Diyanet Vakfı, XLIV.

Baydar, Erkoc T./Ilkilic, İ. (2017): Ethical Evaluation of Euthanasia in the Islamic Tradition, in: Euthanasia and Assisted Suicide, M.J. Cholbi (Ed.), Santa Barbara: ABC-Clio, 147-166.

Baydar, Erkoc Tuba (2017): Fıkhî Açıdan Ötanazi ve Tedavinin Esirgenmesi, Doctoral Dissertation, Marmara University, Institute of Social Sciences.

British Medical Association (2001): Consent, rights and choices in health care for children and young people, London: BMJ Books.

Dörries, Andrea (2003): Der Best-Interest Standard in der Pädiatrie – theoretische Konzeption und klinische Anwendung, in: C. Wiesemann (Ed.), Das Kind als Patient, Frankfurt: Campus, 116-130.

Elmalılı, Muhammed Hamdi Yazır (1942): Hak Dini Kur'ân Dili, Ankara: Diyanet İşleri Reisliği.

Fleischmann, Alan R. (2016): Pediatric Ethics: Protecting the Interests of the Children. Oxford University Press, New York.

Glannon, Walter (2005): Biomedical Ethics, New York: Oxford University Press.

Ibn Manzûr (1997): Lisân al-Arab, Beirut: Dâr al-Ihyâ al-Turath al-Arab.

Ilkilic, Ilhan (2006): Wann endet das menschliche Leben? Das muslimische Todesverständnis und seine medizinethischen Implikationen, in: U.H.J. Körtner (Ed.), Lebensanfang und Lebensende in den Weltreligionen. Beiträge zu einer interkulturellen Medizinethik, Neukirchen-Vlyun: Neukirchener, 165-182.

Ilkilic, Ilhan (2014): End-Of-Life decisions at the beginning of life, in: İ. İlkılıç/ H. Ertin/R. Brömer/H. Zeeb (Eds.), Health, Culture and the Human Body, Istanbul: BETIM Center Press, 433-444.

Ilkilic, Ilhan (2017): Interkulturelle Kompetenz als Schlüsselqualifikation für Gesundheitsberufe, in: Gesundheit Gesellschaft Wissenschaft 17, 24-30.

Isfahanî, Muhammad b. Mufaddal Ragıb (2002): Mufradat al Alfaz al-Qur'an, "al-bala", Damascus: Dâr al-Kalam.

Kutluer, İlhan (1995): "elem", TDV İslam Ansiklopedisi (TDV Encyclopedia of Islam) Istanbul, XI.

Sachedina, A (2009): Islamic Biomedical Ethics: Principles and Application, New York: Oxford University Press.

Sarraj al-Tusî, Abu Nasr Abdullah b. Ali al-Sarraj (1996): Kitab al-Luma fi al-Tasawwuf, translated by Hasan Kâmil Yılmaz, Istanbul: Altınoluk.

Schulz-Baldes, Annette (2006): Therapiebegrenzung in der Neonatologie: Entscheidungen im besten Interesse des Kindes? in: J. Schildmann/U. Fahr/J. Vollm ann (Eds.) Entscheidungen am Lebensende in der modernen Medizin: Ethik, Recht, Ökonomie und Klinik, Berlin: Lit, 87-106.

Snell-Hornby, Mary (2007): Übersetzen, in: J. Straub/A. Weidemann/D. Weidema nn (Eds.), Handbuch interkulturelle Kommunikation und Kompetenz, Stuttgart: J.B. Metzler, 86-94.

Stuhlinger, M. (2005): Das Kindeswohl als zentrale ethische Norm in der Pädiatrie, in: Zeitschrift für Medizinische Ethik 51, 153-165.

Sulamî (1981): Sülemî'nin Risâleleri, translated by Süleyman Ateş, Ankara: Ankara University Publications.

Sulamî, Abu Abd al-Rahman (1981): Tis'at al-Kutub, ed. Süleyman Ateş, Ankara: Ankara University Publications.

Qadî Abd al-Jabbar (2013): Sharh al-Usul al-Hamsa: Mu'tezile'nin Beş İlkesi, translated by, İlyas Celebi, İstanbul: Türkiye Yazma Eserler Kurumu Publications.

PART III

Broadening the View: Narrative-Ethical and Theological Contributions

Uprooted

Towards a Medical Ethics of Suffering

Hille Haker

Introduction

Suffering is the actualization of human vulnerability, which is a fundamental experience in human life; it may be punctual or a state, self-inflicted or inflicted by others, i.e. the result of moral injuries and harms; but it may also be the result of a functional break-down, which may be caused by a disease. Etymologically, the German term "leiden" has its roots in traveling to foreign places, pointing to the risks when encountering the "unknown". Affliction, Simone Weil says, "is an uprooting of life, a more or less attenuated equivalent of death, made irresistibly present to the soul by the attack or immediate apprehension of physical pain" (Weil 1977, 440). When one is severely suffering, one is no longer "at home" in one's body.[1] Suffering is tied to transition, translation and transformation; it is a pathos that threatens the agency and the personhood of oneself (Cassel 2004). Suffering is not a good that can be aimed at; it is an "evil" that an agent strives to avoid; although, paradoxically, suffering is a *Widerfahrnis*, a passive experience beyond the control of the agent, that in first-person narratives is nevertheless often described as transformative in a positive sense.

Medical interventions are but one among several responses to suffering. They rest upon the epistemologies that define medicine as science and clinical practice. Non-medical responses may include the personal narratives of reinterpreting one's life-story (cf. Lindemann Nelson 2001; Frank 1995); social responses may include measures of accommodation aimed at enabling those who are disabled to participate in the social life; religious responses may give suffering a particular meaning, for example, as "redemptive", and they may entail religious rituals and practices.

Both sides of an experience, the pathos or *Widerfahrnis* of suffering and the responses to it by different actors, demonstrate an ethical dimension that requires further scrutiny. The following reflections are an attempt to structure the ethical dimensions of suffering in the context of illness; I begin with the

---

1   Cf. for a thorough analysis in the vein of Heidegger's and Sartre's phenomenology: Svenaeus 2014; Svenaeus 2015.

© BRILL SCHÖNINGH, 2022 | DOI:10.30965/9783657715428_010

medical understanding of health and disease, followed by newer approaches to the phenomenology of illness and suffering. I will then reflect upon responses from what I will call the first-person and the second-person standpoint, and the ethical dimension of these responses, which I will call the responsible responses. I will conclude with some thoughts how a medical ethics of suffering may profit from the insights I have gained in this article.

Health and Disease in Medicine

Since medical inventions and developments in molecular biology and genetics, medical technologies, and pharmacology resulted in radical shifts of medical research and practices, the understanding of health and diseases, too, changed. One of the most influential account of health and disease in the late 20th century was offered by Christopher Boorse in 1977. He has maintained the definition with minor adjustments over the last fifty years, and I will take his recent response to critics as my reference point (Boorse 2014).[2] Boorse's concept, coined by him as "biostatistical theory", represents a naturalistic or objectivist understanding of health and disease. He defines health as the dynamic bodily "normal functional ability: the readiness of each internal part to perform all its normal functions on typical occasions with at least typical efficiency" (Ibid., 684). Disease, over time recoined by Boorse as "[pathology] is a type of internal state which impairs health, i.e., reduces one or more functional abilities below typical efficiency" (Ibid., 684).[3] This concept, Boorse holds, is value-free and theoretical, while other concepts such as "illness" or "disability" are value-laden and hence not compatible with his strictly scientific and theoretical approach. Boorse's understanding represents the epistemological model of medicine today, even when medical professionals are not following him explicitly; it offers a criterion, namely the *substantial deviation* from a state of *normal functioning* that demarcates the non-pathological from the pathological, the normality of function from the pathological "sub-normality of function" in physical or mental states. Addressing his critics, Boorse argues that his understanding of "normal functioning" is not value-laden as some critics have argued; it does not pathologize any difference but serves as the only possible way to describe the conceptual difference between health and disease.[4]

---

2 For a critique from an ethical perspective cf. Bobbert 2000.

3 Boorse agrees with the characterization of "naturalistic" or "objectivist" for his definition.

4 Critics will not be convinced, especially since even as late as 2014, Boorse mentions the functional "abnormality" of homosexuality, arguing that this labeling still does not "pathologize"

Without going into the details of the discussion on the adequacy of the definition, for Boorse the term pathology refers to the (theoretical) study or science of suffering; he is convinced that an objective or naturalist criteriology can be constructed, linking the practical and clinical necessity to distinguish between health and disease to the theoretical research as pathology. As Jeffrey Bishop (Bishop 2012),[5] building on Michel Foucault's studies, has shown, however, this epistemological paradigm must be seen in the historical contexts of Western medicine: the first context concerns the often-described development of medicine as science, beginning in early modernity. With the rise of anatomical studies and with the new technologies since the 19th century that offered radically new insights into organisms, the medical epistemology changes dramatically. Now, the *anticipatory corpse*, Bishop argues, becomes the ultimate, albeit negative model of the dysfunctional body, serving via negativa as the norm for the healthy, functioning living body. The second historical context of medical science is tied to the science of social behavior, also starting in the 17th century and changing again in the 19th century, especially with the invention of the modern tools of statistics; with their help, a generalized notion of "normality" is constructed and reinforced. Today, evidence-based medicine, resting as much on the naturalistic epistemology of the body as functional unity as on the construction of generalized models of behavior is the standard of scientific medical practices. It is used in almost all kinds of Western medical research, and it affects all kinds of medical practice in Western cultures. Whereas the medical sciences are more concerned with the functional side of the body, medical humanities address the psychological, social, and spiritual dimension of suffering, often applying empirical social sciences (Bleakley 2015).[6] Overall, medical humanities, together with medical ethics, emphasize the relevance of the subjective, intersubjective, and transcendent dimensions, which cannot be grasped in a purely naturalistic epistemology. In contrast to medical *interventions*, medical *interactions* depend heavily on the communication between

---

this sexual orientation in his strict understanding of functional impairment of health. This ignores the interdependence of epistemological, medical and social concepts of normality that nobody has brought more to attention than Michel Foucault in his historical studies on "biopower" and "biopolitics".

5 The following reflections stem from a more thorough discussion of Bishop's work (cf. Haker 2016).

6 However, in recent years, ethnographic studies have emerged as a powerful method within the medical humanities, questioning the critical approach Bishop takes towards them. Furthermore, narrative medicine and narrative medical ethics, too, is by now a well-established approach, often used in the education of medical professionals. For a discussion of the emergence of an "empirical ethics" within medical ethics cf. Haker 2015a.

the patients, their families, significant others, and the medical staff. This is why, within the doctor-patient relationship, not only the most basic communication skills matter (for example the skill to transmit information correctly and clearly, or shying away from any directive counseling), but rather, a whole range of skills are required, including the understanding and interpretation of verbal and nonverbal expressions, gestures, facial expressions, especially concerning pain. As I will show below, these skills require more and other competences than the application of one's knowledge of a disease, and more than the ability to transmit medical information. Throughout this essay, I will turn to David Rieff's book, an account of the last two years in the life of his terminally ill mother, Susan Sontag, written from the perspective of her son who was one of her caretakers. I will turn to this book because it is an exceptional text that is highly reflective, yet subjective, a first-person account that I will nevertheless call the second-person standpoint in contrast to the first-person standpoint of a suffering person (Rieff 2008). David Rieff recalls the day his mother received the cancer diagnosis in the early 2000s, which for her is the third time over the course of her life to get this diagnosis. In David Rieff's words,

> Dr. A. was quite clear. From the tests that he had done the previous Friday – blood workups and a bone marrow biopsy – he was in absolutely no doubt that my mother had myelodysplastic syndrome. My mother and I both stared at him blankly. The word meant nothing to either of us. Our befuddlement, his frustration. MDS, he explained, slowly and deliberately, as if he had a family of village idiots sitting in front of him, was a particular lethal form of cancer. [...]
>   Like so many doctors, he spoke to us as if we were children but without the care that a sensible adult takes in choosing what words to use with a child. Instead, he proceeded as if in a lecture hall. Neither my mother nor I interrupted him. (Ibid., 6f.)

"Our befuddlement, his frustration". This is a bitter statement by a witness to this conversation, and Rieff makes it clear over the course of his book that his mother did meet other doctors who did not compensate their own communicative incompetence with merely transmitting medical information, and who did not hide behind the mask of professionalism, avoiding any other communication than one in which they are in control. Rendered dumb *as if* they were "a family of village idiots", and infantilized "as if we were children", *as if* the patient and her family were the audience to a lecture they cannot understand or process, Dr. A. seems to not understand that medical interactions, though radically different from understanding the functions of the human body, still require the same diligence, training, and expertise as the biomedical interventions. Susan Sontag is especially devastated by the recommendation to do nothing and instead wait until the cancer gets worse. Not being able to respond to the *Widerfahrnis* seems to her equivalent to succumbing to death. Rieff recalls finding the Leucemia & Lymphomia Society brochure among his mother's belongings after her death. Reading it after her two-year struggle, he understands that Dr. A only followed a standard procedure. He can feel the disconnect between his mother's experience and the Society's approach, from which he quotes: "When a serious disease [sic] is diagnosed and the physician recommends watchful waiting, patients are sometimes dismayed." (Ibid., 54) Dismay, Rieff comments, is more than a euphemism for the suffering and the death sentence that is associated with the diagnosis of MDS. The same euphemism is reflected in the "coping strategies" and the hope that the brochure upholds. After having gone through the process from diagnosis to the ultimate death of his mother, Rieff's reaction is blunt:

> So admirable in other contexts, here the language of hope becomes grotesque. By mischaracterizing the reality, it inadvertently betrays those it seeks to help by effectively infantilizing them and speaking to them as if they can't see through all that equanimity and poise to the terrible things they are, or soon will be, experiencing. (Ibid., 56f.)

Medical professionals from medical assistants to doctors and nurses who encounter patients, together with those who offer them spiritual or pastoral care, must attend to the ways how to accompany and support patients in their processing of "falling" ill or "being" ill. They need to offer more than the technical-medical support and the transmission of information. Any person who suffers from a disease, i.e. from a particular "dys-functioning" of the body, in Boorse's terminology, still does so as an individual, and not just as a particular case of a general category. And this creates a tension between the third-person scientific approach and the first-person experiential approach that can only be bridged when the doctor (or any other medical professional) understands that he or she is not merely the expert of medical knowledge but also a respondent who must approach a patient from the second-person standpoint. One of the most important 20th century philosophers of hermeneutics, Hans-Georg Gadamer, emphasizes the symbolic value of physicians that goes far beyond the science of medicine:

> The doctor's profession possesses in a certain sense a symbolic value. For the task which confronts the doctor is not one of "making" something but rather one of providing help, of enabling patients to recover their health and to return to their everyday lives. Doctors can never completely entertain the illusion that health is something they simply 'make' or which they fully control. They know that it is not themselves or their abilities but rather nature which they help to victory. (Gadamer 1996, 22)

Rieff echoes the dilemma of the doctor-patient relationship in the final part of his book, coming back to the metaphor of the "infantilizing", asymmetric relationship between a doctor and a patient:

> It is all very well to deride that aspect of the relationship between doctor and patient, to speak of how patronizing or objectifying it is, but I am by no means sure there is a way out of the dilemma or even that more candor from the doctors would have been any sort of improvement. For the sad reality is that without the doctors' power to infantilize, which in this context meant to lull and reassure, not condescend to or lord it over her, my mother would have gone mad months before she died. (Rieff 2008, 136)

I will argue below that the medical professionals can, and indeed should, learn from phenomenology how to respond to the experiential dimension of suffering. Jeffrey Bishop, however, argues that over the years, even the medical humanities – including parts of bioethics – who often claim to *overcome* the reductionist view of the medical sciences, apply exactly the same "objectifying" and "generalizing" models that underlie the medical sciences (Bishop 2011). Seen from the historical perspective, they are at risk to thereby contributing to the further construction of the "normal" and the "pathological" patient (cf. Foucault 1978, 2007). When individual persons, however, are turned into a particular case of the general – from Teilhard de Chardin's seven stages of suffering or Elisabeth Kübler-Ross's stage model of dying to the standards of palliative care in hospices – concepts of care operate with the "average human" as the standard, either pressing the individual into this shape or identifying evermore deviations from the thereby socially-constructed patient.[7] In this context, Bishop is particularly critical of the emergence of "spiritual care", that is often contrasted to a more particular religious pastoral care. When spiritual care is conceived as yet another element of the medical practice that must be rationalized by the same criteria of evidence-based medicine as other kinds of medical knowledge, a sociological, functional understanding of the "spiritual" needs and desires is established.[8] Bishop warns especially that spiritual care

---

7   It comes to no surprise then that medical humanities, for example, discuss the "problem" of the "compliant" and "non-compliant" patient, thereby constructing the "good" patient over against the "bad" one. Patients, it seems, often respond to these expectations, anxious not to fall into the latter category (cf. Hercz and Novak 2013, Parker, Bowman, and Kokanović 2018).

8   Cf., for example, this quote from Kalish's review paper of numerous studies applying spiritual care concepts: "As spiritual care has increasingly been considered an integral component of a healthcare treatment plan, spiritual care practitioners have been encouraged to adopt an evidence-based orientation, just as evidence-based practice is encouraged in every other aspect of healthcare." (Kalish 2012, 242)

could replace the traditional model of "care for the soul" with a model that "generalizes" any need a person might have. Once it does, it perfectly makes sense to quantify this part of healthcare just as any other kind of care for the patient, as one of the study reviewed by Naomi Kalish does: "one-week short-term life review for the enhancement of spiritual well being was effective for providing spiritual well being of terminally ill cancer patients, alleviating psychosocial distress and promoting a 'good death'" (Kalish 2012, 244).

The functional and generalizing models are necessary, but they are not sufficient models for the encounters with suffering persons. As a summarizing statement of this part, let me quote from Eric Cassell's study of suffering:

> In the Birth of the Clinic, Michel Foucault equates the ability of doctors to see the disease below the surface, where laypersons cannot gaze, with the power of medicine. The great advances of the nineteenth century medicine involved the invasion of the body – gazing, to use Foucault's term, into its depts. Opening the body not only revealed it but demonstrated the body's powers – the miraculous complexities of human biology. Opening the body permitted the entrance of science into medicine, and there has followed not only effective knowledge and treatment of disease but amplification of the body's powers. [...]. A central task for the twenty-first century is the discovery of the person – finding the sources of illness within the person, generating a method for the relief of illness from that knowledge and revealing the power within the person as the nineteenth and twentieth centuries have revealed the power of the body. (Cassell 2004, 163)

Finding the sources of illness within the person, and not just within the body, requires to shift the method of the "medical gaze" at the sick *body* to the encounter with the embodied *person*. New approaches promise to do exactly this: they aim to rescue medicine and the medical humanities from their scientific and generalizing gaze, shifting the perspective from the human body to the embodied experience of suffering in and from illness.

The Phenomenology of Suffering in Illness

Phenomenology is the study of the connection between appearances, "phenomena", and consciousness. In distinction to the Kantian transcendental philosophy, phenomenology attends to the "embodied" consciousness: *what* we perceive and experience cannot be separated from the way *how* we experience it, and it is important that self-consciousness does not depart from our embodied self-knowledge. The functioning organism that we call our body is never *only* an object that can be described in scientific or "naturalistic" terms; rather, we *are* our body even when we abstract from this "embodiment", taking our body as an object. The term embodiment refers to this inseparability of self and body, and hence, the study of the perception of phenomena must adhere to this insight. We therefore need not dismiss Boorse's functional definition of health and disease entirely but rather situate it within a range of perspectives towards the embodied self. Because the science of health is not detached from its clinical practice, it is not enough to construct a pathology of bodily functions and the deviation from the normal and pretend it does not have further practical ramifications for the clinical practices. If phenomenology is correct, medicine must begin at a different point, namely with the primary experience of suffering from which the science of suffering, i.e. pathology, can never entirely be abstracted. In other words, the concept of health and disease must be reintegrated into the broader concept of the embodied experience of illness in order to better understand how illness and disease, or suffering and the "pathologies of the body" are correlated. But phenomenology claims not only that it offers important insights into the experience of illness, pain, or suffering; it claims that these experiences elucidate characteristics that go far beyond these particular kinds of experience. In analogy to Bernhard Waldenfels, I will understand experience as the dialectic of *pathos and response* (Waldenfels 2002);[9] the pathos entails an "alienness" *within* oneself, which may well manifest itself as alienation *from* oneself. This phenomenon I will now discern a little further, turning especially to Havi Carel's phenomenology of illness (Carel 2016).

There are multiple traditions within phenomenology. In her recent book on the phenomenology of illness, Havi Carel distinguishes between the schools of transcendental, existential, and hermeneutical phenomenology, each of which takes different paths within phenomenology: Husserl, often seen as the founder of phenomenology, is most interested in the conditions of possibility of cognition, while Heidegger and Sartre, for example, give the encounter of self and world an existential twist. I am most inclined to follow the third tradition that connects the tradition of phenomenology with hermeneutics, as Wilhelm Schapp, student of Husserl, or Paul Ricœur, among others, have done, emphasizing the role of understanding, narrative, and interpretation. For as unique as every individual experience is, it is always "entangled in stories" as Schapp has it: we identify a pain that we feel, for example, as migraine, but in doing so, we perceive it in light of the history of meaning we have learned and that we thereby embody both reflectively and non-reflectively. We may then not only respond to pain in view of modern medicine but also by way of

---

9   Waldenfels does not use the term "dialectic" but I hold that it captures the dynamic nature of pathos and response. For the concept of pathos in the context of "feeling" cf. Waldenfels 2008.

the "folk medicine" (in the context of global medicine often called "indigenous medicine"), entailed in narratives of others as well as in the tradition of practical wisdom. We know that there are mitigating drugs that we can take, and we know that the pain will ultimately pass. Unless chronic and severe, the experience of migraines may well be, as Simone Weil says, an "agony that leaves no trace in the soul" (Weil 1977, 440). In contrast, in severe suffering such as chronic headaches or any other severe form of suffering – affliction, in Weil's terminology – the trace will never leave the "afflicted".

Thanks to a growing school of philosophers who turn to phenomenology in order to describe the experience of illness and suffering, we now have some works that thoroughly analyze the subjective, first-person experience of illness, speaking not only *about* it but *from* it, to take up a good formulation of Waldenfels.[10] With Kay Toombs, Carel describes the experience of (severe) suffering in terms of a loss: the loss of wholeness, certainty, control, the freedom to act, and the familiar world. The disabling of life-sustaining body functions means to be "trapped by routine" of the everyday life movements we normally take for granted, because most of our embodied movements and actions are not reflective but habitual: being able to walk and engaging in a conversation, for example, or to climb the stairway of a plane become obstacles that are unbeknownst to most others.[11] Finitude and death enter one's life as the loss of faith in one's embodied existence. It tears down the mask of one's agency, says Carel, leaving a mark on one's embodied self; it is a breakdown of certainty and trust in one's body, a doubt that invades, exposes the vulnerability, and it threatens one's being-at-home in one's body. The social world changes, too, because encounters with others may be shaped by the social constraints of an illness or a disability, requiring a different kind of recognition of the special needs a person might depend upon than societies, especially autonomy-driven societies as the Western ones are prepared to provide. Because social interactions, spaces, and the organization of time is structured around the "abled persons", the social needs of those who do not meet the standards of

---

10   Carel reflects on her breathlessness or, medically speaking, from chronic obstructive pulmonary disease (COPD) in one of the chapters (Carel 2016, Ch. 5); in addition to discussing the works of Husserl, Heidegger, Merleau-Ponty, or Sartre, she draws more specifically on the work of Kay Toombs who has written about her experience of Multiple Sclerosis (cf. Toombs 1992). Waldenfels gives an example of how speaking from, not merely about an experience philosophically can be achieved: "Just as Walter Benjamin demanded from a good translation that it allows the original text to shine through, one can conceive of an indirect speaking and writing that allows the experiences that befall us and feelings that deal with them to shine through." (Waldenfels 2008, 140)

11   Normal functioning is not only a theoretical concept as Boorse holds but deeply embedded in the habitual structure of behavior, which is socially mediated.

this normality are in fact often misrecognized. But it is not only the others who may have difficulties to encounter the suffering person; they, too, may have difficulties to maintain the equilibrium of their individuality and the equivalence to others, as Arne Vetlesen has called it:

> The taking over of my life and my vitality by bodily pain does not only threaten to isolate me, cause me to feel alone in relation to everything around me. It does not only threaten to restrict the entire world to one single point: pain's nondislodgable reality, that turns the world into a place for pain and nothing else, that makes my pain my world. For when pain, now exclusively a seat of all that causes pain, restricts my existence in the world, I lose the experience of being of equal value with and fully intelligible to other people. From now on it is, on the one hand, me and my pain, and on the other, all the rest, those without pain. The more I merge with my body as a sufferer, the more I slide away from other people and all their projects that *transcend* the body and pain out there in the great big world. (Vetlesen 2004, 29f)

The experience of severe suffering, affliction in Weil's term, "chains down our thoughts" and "uproots" us. The pain of suffering is perhaps the most extreme case of being exposed to one's own vulnerability as the pathos of passivity, affectability and passion. While this vulnerability certainly belongs to the human condition, the metaphors used in connection with severe suffering are strikingly clear: illness is personalized as "intruder"; it "enchains" the self; one transitions from the "kingdom" of the well to the "kingdom" of the ill, as Sontag called it; the "sword of Damocles" is, as Rieff says about his mother's terminal cancer diagnosis, "touching her throat". Religious language expresses the "strike"; the feeling of abandonment and forsakenness by the world and by God, as Psalm 31, for example, does, depicting illness as radical rupture of a person's sense of self. Suffering turns time into an everlasting present, and the space where one dwells as bordering on the abyss of death. Despite all these metaphors, no word *represents* the experience of illness, just as no other experience can be represented in language.[12] Metaphors are therefore at the center of hermeneutical phenomenology – they stand for an epistemology that transcends the metaphysics of representation, but also the critical transcendentalism of Kant: in the face of suffering, the new paradigm of philosophy must begin here, with the experience of the gap between pathos and response.

---

12   The whole point of phenomenology, building upon Kant's critique, is that a simple representation is not possible anyway. But this does not mean that no response is possible. Since expression is a constitutive feature of the "language animal", the loss of expression is indeed equivalent to the loss of one's self (cf. Taylor 2016).

If phenomenology and hermeneutics converge at a certain point, it is necessary to explore the theory of understanding, interpretation, and narration. We know that storytelling is an important part of the social texture that forms some social cohesion; only as narrated experience can the *Widerfahrnis* transition into the web of meaning-giving and meaning-making, rendering it, *as* narration, a part of a shared and shareable history.[13] Before modernity, Walter Benjamin writes, narratives have served as vehicles of practical counseling, as didactic tools to formulate a morale, or, as abstractions and conclusions of experiential knowledge, as proverbial practical wisdom (Benjamin 1999). Modernity, Benjamin claims, may have changed the social role of narratives, and experience may at times result in the collective silence or "poverty" of experience. But certainly narratives have never disappeared as a medium of understanding each other. As there is always and necessarily a gap, the diastasis between the *Widerfahrnis* and the response, there is also a gap between the *pathos* of experience and narration. Yet, narratives are the experiential way by which a suffering person returns to the "world", transforming the non-expressible dimension of suffering into expressions, metaphors, or images that have meaning. Often, the transformation begins with the stammering of the lament, but it may turn into the "small stories"[14] entailed in the metaphors of illness, or transition into the "big" narratives of illness that we may, as Arthur Frank has done, identify as narratives of restitution, chaos, or quest, or, as Hilde Lindemann Nelson has done, as narratives of damaged identities awaiting a narrative repair (Frank 1995; Lindemann Nelson 2001). Subjectivity requires first-person narratives, enabling the self to lend meaning to the pathos of the suffering experience – but also to reconnect with others. This is the reason why the narrative dimension of medical interactions is so important. Just as the treatment through medical interventions is a response, with the person present being replaceable and almost collapsing into a third-person standpoint, listening and attending to the "meaning-making" of patients is, too, a response, however bringing the second-person standpoint by means of interaction, to the forefront.

When diagnosed with the most vicious form of cancer in her life, Susan Sontag begins to search for and study every information she can get a hold of. The dire statistics that are associated with her diagnosis do not escape her, and they are devastating. Yet, she has seen all this before, surviving cancer, against

---

13   The theological term "revelation" echoes this understanding of revealing a truth that *requires* the word to be "real". Similarly, experiences that remain completely inarticulate cannot be grasped cognitively. This is the case with our birth and our death: the one is too "early" to be grasped, the other is too "late" to be narrated.

14   This term was coined by Michael Bamberg (cf. Bamberg 2006; 2008).

all odds, already twice. One of her doctors later comments to David Rieff on his mother's belief at the time of her breast cancer treatment that she would be the exception to the rule:

> Terrible as the statistics were, there's a sense in which Susan was absolutely right. The statistics only get you so far. There are always people on the tail end of the curve. They survive, miraculously, like your mother did with breast cancer. Yes, her prognosis was horrific. But she said, "No, I'm too young and stubborn. I want to go for treatment." Of course, statistically she should have died. But she didn't. She was at the tail end of that curve. (Rieff 2008, 30)

Clinging to the paradigm of science, Sontag bravely claims that she will be – again – the exception to the rule. She thereby reflects a culture that puts much faith in science:

> My mother loved science, and believed in it (as she believed in reason) with a fierce, unwavering tenacity bordering on religiosity. There was a sense in which reason was her religion. She was also always a servant of what she admired, and I am certain that her admiration for science (as a child, the life of Madame Curie had been the first of her models) and above all for physicians helped her maintain her conviction – and again, this, too, was probably an extrapolation from childhood – that somewhere out there was something better than what was at hand, whether the something in question was a new life or a new medical treatment. Soon after she got out of Memorial Sloan-Kettering, she began to search for it. Unreasonable? Probably. But the project of looking itself was immensely strengthening to her ... (Ibid., 31)

Sontag cannot let go of her previous strategy: to fight and to survive against all odds, her son recalls:

> [...] almost until the moment she died, we talked of her survival, of her struggle with cancer, never about her dying. I was not going to raise the subject unless she did. It was her death, not mine. And she did not raise it. To have done so would have been to concede that she might die and what she wanted was survival, not extinction – survival on any terms. To go on living: perhaps that was her way of dying. (Ibid., 17)

Rieff recounts his mother's way to survive: knowing her disease by obtaining all information about it, finding the "right doctors", and following through any possible therapy with "the willingness to undergo any amount of suffering" (Ibid., 39). Carel, together with many others who suffer from chronic illnesses, disabilities, or even terminal illnesses stress that the experience of suffering in illness is never *only* static, and rarely linear, and neither are the responses to it. In other words, the suffering person may re-enter the time of history and respond to the pathos by transforming her self-understanding, the practical arrangements of the everyday life, and the approach to the transcendental categories of life, such as time and space. The response may entail the capability to tell the "unique, individual story of suffering". Regarding illness only from the perspective of the statistical prospects *or* only from the perspective of the time-shattering pathos represents, at least in part, a third-person approach that does not necessarily reflect the experience of the suffering persons hic et nunc. With many others, Carel insists that suffering may well, at least under certain conditions, enable the suffering person to respond in emotional, practical, and narrative terms. Similarly, David Rieff detects in his mother's diaries as well as in her essays the "re-writing" of her own story as a survivor's story in terms of a "rationalization of hope", as he calls it.

> As she construed it, her medical trajectory had gone from lethal diagnosis, to medical pessimism, to the search for doctors who did have hope to hold out [...] to agonizing but nonetheless potentially lifesaving treatments, to cure. You did not give in to cancer, you fought it, and if you fought hard enough and, above all, intelligently enough, there was a chance that you could win. (Ibid., 91f.)

While the transformation of suffering may follow a scheme, this certainly does not happen with necessity. Reflecting upon this narrative, Rieff summarizes his mother's response to her illness like this: "keep strong, keep going, keep writing". First-person narratives often show that patients do indeed say that adjustments and accommodations are possible; strength and resilience may be discovered – but no *illness* story can be taken as representative, or as a particular case of a general pattern, even when the biological – and even the statistical – progression or prognosis of a *disease* can be generalized. For some, illness may not exclude what Carel calls a "hedonic adaptation", finding well-being and happiness in one's life – but without attending to the individual experience, such a statement may easily become "grotesque", as Rieff described the tone of false hope in the medical brochure he finds after his mother's death. Carel cites studies that show that chronically ill persons and persons with disability do not self-ascribe a lower level of well-being and happiness than persons who are healthy (cf. Carel 2016, 130-149). Still, since empirical studies imply that there is no significant difference between "healthy" and "ill" persons regarding their well-being, these findings question the assumption that suffering from (and in) illness (or disability) is incompatible with having a "good life". In fact, Carel argues, it is often not the chronically ill or "disabled" persons who define their identity entirely in relation to their illness; others, however, do, especially the more remote they are, to wit speaking of *disease* from the third-person standpoint. This standpoint differs strikingly from the first-person and second-person standpoint, elucidating the risk of detaching the understanding of disease too far from the experiential understanding of *illness*.

With the reception of feminist care ethics, the communitarian philosopher Alasdair MacIntyre tried to shift the focus of ethics from its primary value of autonomy to the acknowledgment of relationality as dependency and interdependency (MacIntyre 1999). MacIntyre shows that the social nature of human beings does not contradict the Aristotelian concept of eudaimonia or self-fulfillment but that this deeper understanding of "well-being" and "happiness" emerges exactly within the "boundaries" of inter-dependency. The second-person standpoint highlights the "social" nature of human beings who are necessarily related to others, and most importantly, related to those others who are most "significant" for the suffering person. Suffering exposes human beings, the "dependent rational animals", to their anthropological or ontological vulnerability. For human beings who are dependent on others to survive, cultures and communities are ways of reducing the risks of the environment and, among others, the vulnerability as susceptibility to suffering. But with Schapp, I want to maintain that suffering also reveals that we are "entangled in stories": if consciousness is tied to the social and historical frames of understanding and intelligibility, the interactions with others are an important part of how one's responses are shaped and articulated. I follow the hermeneutic tradition within phenomenology in part *because* the "self" is never alone and never invents the "script" for the narratives apart from a context of meaning. The social dimension of the self is not a secondary dimension that follows the state of personhood but, to the contrary, it is its primary occasion. Ricœur rightly emphasizes that the capabilities to speak, to act, to narrate, and to respond to others all emerge from and within the social, cultural, and historical contexts of inter-acting with others.[15]

The phenomenology of suffering warns us not to brush over the uprooting of a person in suffering, and this must not be taken lightly. But as we have seen, suffering from/in illness may also confront us with a paradox, namely that suffering does not necessarily linger as the radical pathos as which it is often described. States of chronic illness or disability, we have seen, may also not

---

15   This is how Ricœur describes what he calls the "cabable human" (Ricoeur 2005) – it is a concept of agency that is deeply "entangled" with the actions, lives, and stories of others. Drawing upon her mother-infant studies, Jessica Benjamin has suggested to attend to the pre-reflective inter-agency, questioning thereby a narrow understanding of action as self-conscious and intentional. Her model of "attunement" between inter-agents who are often in asymmetric relations may also be valuable for the multiple asymmetric relations in the context of healthcare, and the necessary attunement in interactions that goes beyond the requirement of cognitive consent-giving (cf. Benjamin 1988, 2017).

contradict happiness and well-being. In a culture that emphasizes autonomy as control over one's body, it is difficult to acknowledge this transformation within the experience of suffering – a paradox that applies also to the concept of dependency and vulnerability. Vulnerability makes human beings susceptible to pain, suffering, and harm, but it is also the condition for the most basic openness to the world, the "affectability" by others (Haker 2018).[16] Like Erinn Gilson, Pamela Sue Anderson stresses that "[s]triving for invulnerability puts us at risk. And it misses the opportunity that vulnerability can offer" (Anderson 2016).

> Vulnerability colours a deeply shared dimension of our lives together as human beings. Failing to recognize and accept this vulnerability can, ironically, leave us open to even greater hurt and loss. (Ibid.)

Emmanuel Levinas has shifted the focus of phenomenology from the self-centered subject of experience to the ethical concept of responsibility for the other.[17] Unlike in other approaches, for him, the self-other relationship is not merely understood in terms of intersubjectivity and sociality. Against Heidegger's "existential" analysis of *Dasein* of existence, which owes much to Kierkegaard's analyses, no other philosopher has argued more radically for the necessity to shift the focus from an ontological to an ethical understanding within phenomenology than Levinas, echoed in his phrase "otherwise than being" (Levinas, 1998, Levinas 1969).[18] Levinas is best known for his ethics of responsibility, which never ceases to reflect upon the infinity that prevents the other from being captured in "experience", language, or knowledge. It is important to note that the path towards responsibility begins with the response to the other, befalling the self – a *Widerfahrnis* and pathos – in the experience of

---

16   Erinn Gilson distinguishes between ontological and situational vulnerability, the latter referring to the particular forms of experiences and states of vulnerability (Gilson 2014). In Haker 2015b I have called the "ontological" vulnerability "anthropological" to stress its connection to the conditio humana; in order to create a more common language, I now take up Gilson's term (cf. Haker 2018).

17   This does not mean, of course, that other phenomenologists have not attended to the self-other relationship. It only means that Levinas shifts phenomenology from ontology to ethics, to understand the self strictly from this encounter. For a discussion of the "other" in the phenomenological tradition cf. the seminal study by Michael Theunissen (Theunissen 1984).

18   Levinas counters Heidegger's claim that human existence, "Dasein", means the "being towards death". "Death in Heidegger is an event of freedom, whereas for me the subject seems to reach the limit of the possible in suffering. It finds itself enchained, overwhelmed, and in some way passive. Death is in this sense the limit of idealism." (Levinas 1987, 71) For a more thorough analysis cf. Haker 2005.

the other's vulnerability, captured in the "nakedness" of the face. The Hebrew language, which Levinas evokes with this term, understands *"panim"* as a pars pro toto for the embodied self, undermining the dualism of body and soul of the ancient Greek tradition. The face exposes humans to each other, rendering them impressionable, affectable – and vulnerable to each other. The encounter with the other is therefore necessarily an encounter with a *vulnerable* other. Adding another layer to the pathos of suffering, namely the lack of agency as lack of responsibility, Levinas stresses that suffering transforms a person into the "state of irresponsibility, the infantile shaking of sobbing" (Levinas 1987, 72). Encountering an other in this state means that in the self-other relation, the intrasubjective dialectic of pathos and response is duplicated or "doubled" in the *intersubjective* interaction, captured in the *ethical* dynamic of a "call and response". Suffering, Levinas holds, only radicalizes what underlies *any* experience between the self and the other:

> Someone who expresses himself in his nudity – the face – is one to the point of appealing to me, of placing himself under my responsibility: Henceforth, I have to respond for him ... The other individuates me in the responsibility I have for him. (Levinas 2000, 12)

Sontag's metaphor of the "sword of Damocles that touches her throat" is a metaphor of the anticipation of death. David Rieff's reflections demonstrate that death was indeed constantly present for both his mother and himself; it is present as the wound, a "reminder" of the future, which comes closer and closer until the moment of death arrives. The most touching parts of Rieff's essay concern his reflections on his own position, the second-person standpoint in relation to his mother. His account is therefore an invaluable source for a phenomenology of compassion that must complement the phenomenology of suffering.

Accompanying his mother in her terminal illness, Rieff is often conflicted about his own responses to his mother's suffering. Ultimately, his book is therefore an account of his own compassion, a son's suffering – with his mother.[19] Often, he recalls, he was at a loss of words himself, overwhelmed by the *pathos* of the experience to watch his mother suffer. This is how he describes his own state of mind:

---

19   "Obviously, there is no comparison between the sufferings of a person who is ill and the sufferings of those who love them. But I think there is something similar about the helplessness you feel as a friend or a relative." (Rieff, 2008, 80f.)

I answered as best I could. What I mean by this is that I gave the answers that I believed she wanted to hear, the answers that would give her the strength to go on. And it was so clear that what she wanted to hear was good news and nothing else. Of course, sometimes even giving the right answer did not pierce her despair. I think I did right. But I did it ineptly. Inside, I was shutting down, almost as if, instinctively, I realized that I could not handle my own emotion as well as hers, as if also I could not tell her these things and be aware of myself enough to know whether or not I myself believed them. At the time, this shutting down seemed like an inevitable choice. Looking back, though, I am by no means sure it was the right one. (Rieff 2008, 98f.)

The ultimate question Rieff wrestles with is: What *is* a responsible response to a suffering person?

Towards an Ethics of Suffering: Compassion and Consolation

Summarizing my argument so far, I want to keep the following thoughts in play: first, suffering from and/or in illness is one experience of suffering, rooted in the vulnerability of human beings. Nobody, I believe, doubts that the medical approach must be re-connected to the experience of illness, because without the trust of patients in medical practices and the professionals who conduct them it is impossible to mitigate the suffering; the question is whether and how that is possible within the current Western medical system. Second, the phenomenology of suffering has shown that *patients* themselves respond to their suffering, and they do so in multiple ways that may or may not follow a generalized, yet culturally mediated "script". Responses differ from patient to patient, and they differ over time, too. The first-person standpoint is, however, intertwined with the second-person standpoint, and their encounter is thereby framed in terms of responsibility. The question now is whether we can discern the responsibility of those who accompany patients more distinctly in ethical terms.

Suffering calls for a specific response – a *moral* response that resonates with Levinas' formulation of the other "placing himself under my responsibility". While there is an ongoing debate between philosophy of mind and phenomenology whether and in what way we have "access" to another's mind or how we experience the other,[20] suffice it to say that the responsible response to a suffering person is not a self-centered or world-exploring experience but a response to an other whom one *cares* about. In his work on empathy and sympathy,

---

20   Cf. for a concise discussion of the debate Zahavi 2014a and his own phenomenological theory of intersubjectivity Zahavi 2014b.

Scheler, Zahavi argues, understands that the *Fremdwahrnehmung* or perception of other minds (as the German term is, unfortunately, translated) occurs without the detour through the first-person memory ("I know how you suffer, because I have experienced the same") or through imagination of the other's suffering – memory and imagination may *accompany* sympathy, but they are not the constitutive elements of it. For Scheler, in sympathy the *perception* and the *concern* for the other coincide (Zahavi 2014a). Levinas, following Scheler in this point, argues that in the encounter with the other, the solitary self is *ruptured*. Compassion is therefore neither the recognition of one's own past or imagined suffering in the other nor the experience of the other's suffering in one's own body. Rather, it is the experience of the other *as* sobbing, squirming, groaning. In a similar vein, Martha Nussbaum reminds us that compassion is not about oneself:

> For if it is to be for another, and not for oneself, that one feels compassion, one must be aware both of the bad lot of the sufferer and of the fact that it is, right now, not one's own. If one really had the experience of feeling the pain in one's own body, then one would precisely have failed to comprehend the pain of another *as other*. (Nussbaum 2001, 327)

The suffering of a person may always be opaque and obscure for a second person, requiring patience and thorough attention, but to be an experience of compassion or sympathy, perception and concern for the other must converge – even though, as Weil warns us, compassion with the "afflicted" may not be the norm but rather the exception – a "miracle", as she has it, because affliction cannot be communicated or shared: "Compassion for the afflicted is an impossibility. When compassion truly produces itself, it is a miracle more astonishing than walking on water, healing the sick or even the resurrection of the dead." (Weil 1977, 441)

Ironically, the debate on compassion or empathy, especially in the philosophy of mind, centers so much on the discernment of cognition that the suffering other is once more pushed to background. Hence, rather than concentrating on this discourse, I want to focus instead on another aspect that brings us closer to the ethical realm. In his work on philosophical anthropology, the German philosopher Hans Blumenberg describes the phenomenon of consolation as an anthropological capability that reveals the paradox of suffering in yet another way, now in relation to the other (Blumenberg 2006).[21] It adds to the insight that vulnerability, the susceptibility to illness, harms, and structural injustice is at the same time the condition for our openness

---

21   For a more thorough interpretation cf. Haker (2015b).

to be affected by others at all. Blumenberg holds that even though nothing and nobody can *undo* the suffering, human beings are still capable of being comforted or consoled by others. Note that this capability is not an effective action – a good that one strives for and sets out to achieve – but rather an authorization of *another* person. Blumenberg calls it a delegation. Connecting it to the human condition of vulnerability, this delegation of one's suffering to the other can be discerned further: it reflects the fundamental trust that one can be *affected positively* by others. Trust is necessary in order to take the "risk" of opening to the other and as such the undercurrent of the capability to be comforted (Bernstein 2015, 2011). Compassion and comfort, we can now understand, are connected to responsibility, because responding responsibly means, in the most fundamental way, that the second-person does not betray the trust of the suffering person who places not only her body but herself under the other's (and others') responsibility.

Consolation entails the paradox of responding when no response seems possible. But there is no easy way from compassion to consolation – and sometimes, there is perhaps no way, just the silence and the failing words of those who know that they are the ones who should speak, yet have no words themselves. This is what David Rieff says about the impossibility to comfort:

> Looking back, I wonder if there is any silence worse than the silence of the sick room. It is the silence of that horror-stricken intuition that in a cancer ward, at least, the real and the catastrophic are often one and the same. And of course it is also the silence of impotence, of the powerlessness of feeling to change anything, of the vanity of human wishes. You find yourself hoping, and yet you know there is no empirical basis for such hope. The words form, but fail to emerge when you open your mouth. In your head, there is a voice screaming, "Say something, do something!" But there is nothing to do and everything that seems possible to say, at least to someone who wants to be reassured of something that you don't have the basis to reassure them of, either has no bearing on what is really going on or involves you in pure fable making – a species of nannyspeak. In effect, you find yourself saying a slightly more sophisticated version of "there, there, it will be all right." But that is a lie. It will not be all right [...] as somewhere you know perfectly well, no matter how much you deny it to yourself or others, or even set about intubating yourself psychologically to the point where you don't even think it at three in the morning. (Rieff 2008, 133f.)

Yet, the "there, there, it will be all right" does perhaps more than Rieff can acknowledge. Taking up the burden means, first and foremost, to be *present*, to be-there-with-the-other, as Jeffrey Bishop calls it. The dialectic of pathos and response takes place on both sides, though the "pathos" of compassion is not identical with the pathos of suffering. Bishop emphasizes, correctly in my view, that "the response to suffering is a suffering-with-the-other and undergoing-with-the-other" (Bishop 2011, 304). Compassion and consolation are connected to the ethical stance of responsibility, I said. But suffering and comfort are connected through the concept of compassion, which constitutes the *interpersonal* relation of care and concern for the other that affects the second-person as well as the first-person. Though perhaps a little too emphatically embracing the language of the gift, Bishop emphasizes the reciprocal "giving" and "receiving" that marks any interpersonal relation:

> The response is not an altruistic response, in which the responder receives nothing, for she has already received the call to being-there-with, a call that constitutes her purpose for being. The call changes the perceiver, even if she cannot respond. The call changes the receiver, if it is gladly received. However painful, if the call is received, it is gift. [...] being-there-with-the-suffering-other changes the way that each is embodied. (Bishop 2011, 304)

I believe that this insight captures what Levinas means by the rupture of the solitary self in the encounter with the other. One should note that this is a much more radical reversal of the ethics of autonomy than merely pointing to the interdependence, as MacIntyres does: Levinas argues that the second-person is constituted as a moral self in the compassion with the other: in the coincidence of the perception of the other and the care and concern for her. A person's agency does not primarily originate from one's self-consciousness or the capability to act according to reason; neither is it simply embedded in a web of interdependence. A person's agency, in its full meaning of response-ability, is provoked by the other, and when it is received, it "constitutes her purpose for being", as Bishop says in the quote above.[22]

In combination with Bishop's formulation, i.e. "being-with-the-other" and "undergoing-with-the-other", we can now discern compassion and consolation as the first responses to the first-person experience of suffering, as responses from the second-person standpoint; they are *responsible* responses when the act of being present-with-the-other in the experience of suffering acknowledges not only the vulnerability of the other but also the tremendous trust that the "delegation" of suffering entails. In other words, the gift that the second person receives is not so much "the call to being-there-with" but in the first

---

22   This is a thought that was already emphasized by Fichte who called it the "summons" of the self through the Other, and it plays an important role in the concept of recognition. In his study on recognition, Paul Ricœur points to the concept of "gift giving" and "gift receiving" as an alternative to the Hegelian struggle for recognition. Interestingly, it remains closely connected to the concept of responsibility, which Ricœur, in contrast to Levinas, does not only understand as a response but also as imputability or accountability (Ricœur 2015).

instance, it is the suffering person's *trust* that the second-person will indeed perceive her with care and concern. And lest we forget: the structure of the encounter with a suffering person is ultimately *not* based on the reciprocity that underlies any gift exchange or, for that matter, recognition. It is based on the asymmetrical compassion as the *ethical* understanding of the care and concern for the other. Levinas is right: the "call" to respond is not only an appeal; it is at the same time a "summons" that charges the response-able agent with the *duty* to respond. We can now see that Blumenberg's concept, the capability to delegate one's suffering, is at the same time, an ethical endowment of trust, the "entrustment" of oneself to the other, *and* a charge, namely that the response-able agent may act responsibly and not *betray* this trust. The delegation may therefore be seen from more than one angle: it is the suffering person's first step out of the "bare" pathos, trusting to be affected positively by the other and being supported; it is a gift to the other that *endows* him or her with trust; but from the second-person's perspective, it is also a summons that obligates.

So far, I have not even raised the question what responsibility really entails in practical terms. We may understand that the medical interventions rest upon a third-person standpoint, focusing on the suffering body, pain, and all kinds of treatments and therapies. This is certainly necessary and therefore responsible in the context of suffering from an illness. I have explained the second-person standpoint as an experiential response to the first-person's suffering, and I have identified the ethical dimension of the "response" by way of the gift giving and gift receiving, by way of trusting and being trusted, and by way of the summons that reveals the normative dimension of the self-other relation. As soon as (or as long as) the suffering person finds a thread that leads her out of the darkness of silence, the intertwining of self and other is maintained. But what if the wishes of the suffering are unjustified from the second-person standpoint (and, perhaps, from the third-person standpoint, too)? David Rieff, for example, is not convinced that his mother's "narrative", summarized as "try everything medically possible, no matter how much you suffer" is adequate and whether he, in turn, should not have countered her narrative with another one, one that would have enabled her to accept her death better. However, as we have seen, he cannot come up with *any* narrative that would have been able to take away the pain of death:

> [...] in the end, those of us who loved her failed her as the living always fail the dying, for we could not actually do the only thing she really wanted, which was to stave off extinction for just some time longer, let alone give her what I'm afraid is all too accurately called a new lease on life. Only her doctors could do that. So she clung to them, as a shipwrecked sailor to a spar, for as long as she possibly could [...]. (Rieff 2008, 136)

Susan Sontag found doctors who followed through with her, offering her experimental or risky cancer treatments. Yet, in the process, Rieff, says, "it was not only his mother who was stripped of her dignity" (ibid.). The "aggressive" medical response that Sontag wanted and received is not uncontested even in the medical profession. Rieff recounts a conversation with a doctor, Diane Meyer, who is a pioneer in the US for palliative care for terminally ill persons. Her view differs strikingly from her colleague – and from Sontag's:

> "It's so difficult," she said. "As a physician, you don't want to impose your quantitative, Cartesian view of probabilities on an individual person who says, 'That's probabilities, that's not me. I'm a fighter. I want that thousand to one chance and who are you to say that it's not worth it?' Whose life is it anyway? The result is that, as doctors, we end up through that kind of thinking becoming unwitting participants in a folie à deux with patients and family of caving to the desire to live, because it is respectful of the patient and who she or he is and their perception of the right way to live, while realizing, in the other part of your brain, that there's essentially no chance that this is going to help, that it's definitely going to cause harm and side effects, that it's hugely expensive out of the public trough, and it is a very wearing kind of cognitive dissonance." (Ibid., 113f)

Meyers poses a question that resonates well in a culture that values autonomy as the highest good: "Whose life is it anyway?" And yet, does acknowledging the uniqueness of the experience of suffering mean that we can isolate and abstract the responses from the relations and contexts of acting? Sontag's desire to try any therapy that is possibly available still requires the medical assessment by her doctors. Rieff does not say that he himself had any professional support in his role as the second-person – he says that he could only shut off his own suffering in the process. Rieff says his mother could not reconcile with her death, and all the love she received did not console her. The only thing that helped her was her doctor's assurance to medically try whatever he could to make her survive. "In retrospect, though, I realize that, obsessed with death as she was, this positive denial was at a deep level the denial of death itself." (Ibid., 92) But this denial is far from a singular or "unprecedented" response to the pathos of a terminal illness: rather, it is inscribed into current Western cultures, nurtured by the "medical gaze" and the progress narrative that constructs its own telos, to wit to "fix" the dysfunctional body and to overcome, ultimately, any human suffering and, perhaps, even the human condition of mortality, as *google* director Ray Kurzweil predicts (Friend 2017). This is the one extreme to respond to the pathos of suffering – and one that requires a critical ethical evaluation.

Often, this cultural narrative is countered by the implicit and explicit ethics of hospice care that draws much from the Christian religious tradition from which it originates. But more often than not, hospice care is caught between

Scylla and Charybdis: Either it follows the "script" of evidence-based medical care that cannot capture the depth of "uprooting" that suffering and death means for the living, or it follows a religious "grand narrative" that links suffering to some kind of divine providence: Maybe it is sin that has caused suffering? Maybe it is a divine punishment, a test, a spiritual purification, or the sanctification of the self? In its long history, Christianity has created many narratives concerning suffering, but the connection of suffering as condition for the encounter of God is a consistent trope.[23] One example may suffice as an example of this belief, echoed and often amplified in Christian theology. Merry quotes from A. Elchaninov, The Diary of a Russian Priest:

> Illness [...] has confirmed me even more deeply in the conviction that if a man is with Christ, then he is with suffering, and that there is no other way for the Christian than the way of pain, inward and outward. (Merry 2004, 78)

While the search for immortality represses suffering and death, this theological approach seeks suffering as pathway to redemption. Like its counterpart, it requires a critical ethical evaluation, however this time from a more decidedly theological perspective. According to this understanding, suffering is "the way to be with" God, and even though God may not *wish* our suffering, he [sic] – the omnipotent and omniscient Divine power – nevertheless lets it happen. Hence, the evil of suffering is, ultimately, transformed into a good, either as a moral transformation of a sinner or the sanctification of a human being by God. Rather than attending to the contexts and experiences of the suffering persons, theological accounts of suffering often center the theological question on the justification and justice of God in the face of suffering, or theodicy. Like the pathology in medical science, theology, too, does not begin with the phenomenology of suffering; the experiential dimension is pushed to the background, because suffering is a necessary evil, a means to achieve the good of "spiritual healing", just as in medicine the pain of therapies is the necessary evil to achieve the good of the medical cure. In many religious traditions, prayer is seen as an important pathway to healing (and forgiveness), complemented, in the Catholic tradition, by the sacraments.[24] In spiritual care concepts, the theology of "purification" is transformed into the language of a secularized,

---

23   For a concise overview from a theological-hermeneutical perspective cf. Merry 2004.

24   Merry quotes from the sacramental rite of healing: Part of the rite from the 8th century reads, "let it [the oil] do away with all suffering, every defilement of flesh or spirit, and every evil, so that in this, too, your most holy name may be glorified (...)" (Merry 2004, 80), quoting from A. Strittmatter, "The Barberinium S. Marci of Jacques Goar," (Ephemerides Liturgicae, Rome, 1993, p. 226).

interreligious and therefore pluralistic culture; yet, it is echoed when suffering becomes the occasion to *restitute* one's balance, to *reconcile* with one's life, or to *re-evaluate* the deeds and values of one's life. In the context of end of life care and hospice, these life evaluations become life *reviews*, shifting the focus from the prospective orientation to a retrospective reflection (Flanagan 2017).

The tradition of mysticism bears perhaps the most radical expression of suffering, to wit as *self-sacrifice* on the way to encounter God. All these theological tropes run through the long history of Christian theology. Let us turn, once again, to Simone Weil, certainly not immune to the self-sacrificial love of God Weil speaks of severe suffering in terms of affliction: affliction, she says, taking Job as an example, results in the absence of God, an abandonment that equals death:

> Affliction causes God to be absent for a time, more absent than a dead man, more absent than light in the utter darkness of a cell. What is terrible that if, in this darkness where there is nothing to love, the soul ceases to love, God's absence becomes final. (Weil 1977, 442)

Weil's interpretation of the crucifixion follows this vein, but now, the distance and abandonment occurs no longer between a human being and God but between God and God, a "tearing apart" of the One: Nothing, she notes, could be further from God than the Crucified – and yet, they belong together in the "bond of the supreme union":

> This tearing apart, over which supreme love places the bond of the supreme union, echoes perpetually across the universe to the depths of silence, like two notes separated and merging, like a pure and heartbreaking harmony. This is the Word of God. The whole entire creation is only a vibration. (Weil 1977, 444)

Human suffering or affliction, understood in analogy to the abandonment of God by God in the "depth of silence", renders suffering a part of God's own suffering, one note in the music of creation, its "pure and heartbreaking harmony". Sin is irrelevant to this thought: Sin, Weil holds, is not a distance. Echoing Augustine and the long tradition of equating sin with human freedom, sin is merely a "turning of our eyes in the wrong direction". Affliction, in contrast, does not come with a rationale of that sort; it resembles the *tohu-wabohu* of chaos and disorder that somehow is not completely undone in creation. Weil's metaphors are striking: affliction is pathos by "chance", driven by a "blind mechanism", not a purpose; it is a "metallic chill"; it tosses some people around, "freezing" all those it touches, flinging them at the symbolic foot of the Cross, the ultimate "depth of silence". Affliction is not only not sin, affliction is also not martyrdom: "Christ was afflicted. He did not die like a martyr. He died like a common criminal, in the same class as thieves, only a little more ridiculous. For affliction is ridiculous." (Weil 1977, 445) In this theological interpretation, we find metaphors that function as placeholders for one possible narrative within theology; Weil's expression resemble those that are used in phenomenological accounts, now inscribed into theology. Again, we encounter the paradox that is echoed in almost all narratives of suffering: in the midst of abandonment, which is the absence of love, language, and relation, exactly these: love, language, and relation are found. In the words of St. Paul, at the heart of the Christian religion, we encounter the "folly of God" (1 Corinthians, 1, 25). For Weil, understanding affliction in this way enables humans to love God, to *hand themselves over to God*, which is another expression for the "endowment" with a gift. Faith therefore echoes the trust that is the condition of opening oneself up to the other, only that in faith, it is the opening to God.

Following Weil in the separation of affliction and sin, it appears more than problematic to seek a cause of suffering, be it in a person's wrongdoing or in divine providence.[25] Connecting suffering, especially suffering from illness, with sin is itself a sin, as the story of Job warns. But because this narrative is so pervasive, it is the task of theological ethics to *reveal, critique, and correct* it and instead help those who suffer, and those who are-with-the-suffering in compassion, to understand that this response – expressed either by the suffering person herself or the second-person respondent – is, in fact, not Christian at all. Reconciliation with death cannot mean to add harm to one's own or another person's suffering – it is as irresponsible a response as the false promise that science will be able to overcome suffering and death. Theological ethics must reassure those who do not know how to respond that there may be a return to language, love, and relation. It must reassure those who do not know how to respond, that compassion entails the patience to wait for the authorization to act – and to abstain from action if the suffering is not ready to "delegate" her suffering to the other. Theologically speaking, and in contrast to the interpretation of an *intentional* abandonment of a suffering human being by God, the mystery of God is that even in the depth of silence, in the diastasis or gap between the pathos and the response, God is still – or already – present. According to the Gospel narratives of the crucifixion, Jesus' last word is *not* about abandonment. It is exactly the opposite. Quoting Psalm 31, the

---

25   This does not mean that suffering can never be an effect of one's wrongdoing – but as a trope for suffering in illness it is inappropriate; it resembles the assertion that the victim of harm (by others) must somehow have caused her victimization – or that it was God's will. In both incidents, the rationalization of suffering is itself harmful.

torture-stricken, dying Jesus *entrusts* (the Hebrew word is *paqad*) his spirit (the Hebrew word *ruach* means the breath of life, another pars pro toto for the whole person), into the hands of God. All one may hope for is that a suffering person may say and do the same.

Conclusion

Nothing in this essay gives us a clear understanding of the right or wrong responses to suffering, whether it is regarding the suffering self or the second-person standpoint. Though we have norms, they require the practical reason that ethics, the theoretical reflection on moral judgments and lived morality, embraces. Here, I want to only draw some conclusions that are meant to pave the way to an ethics of suffering that builds upon the insights I have explored.

First and over against a certain reading of the Christian tradition, suffering is not a good that human beings strive for or should strive for; ethically speaking, it has no value and cannot be regarded as instrumental to the good life. As part of the human condition, i.e. vulnerability as the susceptibility to suffering, suffering is unavoidable. Moral harm, in contrast, is different from chance: It is based on intentional action, purposefully inflicting a wound to the other. Moral harm is the failure to respond responsibly to the other, and the suffering resulting from it must be accounted for. As such, it is an injustice that cannot be a feature of the just God.[26]

Second, virtue ethics, now often called the ethics of the good life, is one entry point to reflect upon suffering more distinctly in an ethical way. I understand this dimension of ethics to be a hermeneutical ethics (Haker 2010; Mieth 2002). Reading the tradition of ethics, from the biblical wisdom literature to the Stoic, Aristotelian, medieval or contemporary virtue ethics creates opportunities to practice the "work" of self-formation – and possible transformations – in relation with others. In the encounter with the different cultures of the theological tradition and different religious traditions, different value systems, and plural narratives of suffering, a hermeneutical ethics offers us an orientation how to practice understanding, how to move between the plural understandings of different traditions while forming a self-identity. Though I will not argue for it here, this must be conceived in terms of a *critical hermeneutical ethics* rather than, as the phenomenological tradition of Heidegger and Gadamer does, in

---

26   This is the reason why Metz, for example, insists that theodicy cannot be given up as a theological trope. It has nothing to do with God's "permission" that suffering happens and everything to do with the justice-seeking God.

terms of an ontological hermeneutics.[27] Even though I referred to the traditional practical wisdom, mediated by storytelling, virtues and norms that ori-
ent our actions and conduct are never *merely* trans-mitted or trans-lated from
one person/tradition to another: the meaning of texts or traditions does not,
ultimately, rest upon an ontological theory of being, just as ethical norms do
not, ultimately, rest upon a metaphysical order of the good. It is the task of a
critical hermeneutical ethics to foster the understanding that self-formation
(or the formation of convictions and dispositions to act) requires more than
an "obedient" reception of the tradition; it requires critique as part of practical
reasoning (Dussel 2014; Ricœur 1998). In this vein, both "grand narratives" that
I have discerned above, the grand narrative of the quest for immortality, and
the grand narrative of punishment, purification, and sanctification through
suffering must be critizised. Furthermore, Dietmar Mieth's understanding of
Narrative Ethics as part of a broader *Modellethik*, which serves as a laboratory
for practical reason, may be used to explore the ethics of suffering as part of a
critical medical Modellethik.

Third, regarding the suffering of others, I believe that the concept of compassion and consolation could be further spelled out in relation to an ethics of
(medical, interpersonal, and pastoral) care. It is closely linked to the teleological ethics or ethics of the good life, pursuing the self-fulfillment or well-being
of the other (and oneself) insofar as a given condition renders this possible.
Here, the phenomenological-ethical understanding that I have offered is indispensable. But compassion, care and concern, or more distinctly consolation
are not only to be seen from the perspective of an ethics of the good life. They
all create the link between the hermeneutical *phenomenology* of the "response"
and the *ethics* of responsibility, which I indeed regard first and foremost in
terms of the care and concern for the other. Care ethics, I hold, stands at the
threshold between teleological ethics and deontological ethics, i.e. the ethics
of duties and moral norms. It may be understood in view of medical care and
cure, nursing and practical support services, but also as the "care for the soul",
as in healthcare chaplaincy. As we have seen, in this context second-person
narratives are as important as first-person narratives for the understanding of
suffering. Together, they create the space for conversation and discernment, as
yet another laboratory for an experiential ethics.

Fourth, in view of normative ethics, the question of what is the "required"
and "just" concern and care paves the way to the deontological dimension
within ethics (Kittay 2016). The principles of medical ethics are necessary

---

27   Cf. for an argument for an ontological hermeneutics Gadamer 1975; Haker 1999; Haker
      2015a.

reference points. If the language of responsibility entails the "summons" of the self by the other, it is crucial to have criteria of the scope and limits of this responsibility. But while we can name abstract principles, such as respect for the patient, the duty not to harm, the care for the patient's well-being, non-discrimination between patients and patient groups, and justice as the overall principle for political and social ethics, these must be discerned and prioritized in the contexts in which the questions of responsibility occur. Moral *understanding* is indeed linked to moral *judgments*, but both are dependent on the "materiality" of the contexts of experiences, constellations, social and legal structures.

Fifth, theological ethics is in a good position to contribute to an ethics of suffering – on the one hand, because there are so many religious residues in Western cultures, even when their medical practices seem to be predominantly secular, and on the other hand because theology is needed as a critique of religious and non-religious metaphors, imageries, narratives, or "grand narratives" that may well add moral injuries to the persons' suffering: if that is the case, these practices, e.g. those labeled as "spiritual healing" must be scrutinized in view of the principles of non-maleficence and beneficence. I have given some hints how the Christian tradition has long contributed to the connection of suffering and sin, exploiting the weakness of suffering persons for practices that do not withstand ethical scrutiny. Regarding the theological trope of providence in the context of medicine and science, theology must not only critique the imagery of the un-empathic God, mocking humans just like the humans mocked the crucified Jesus, the Son of Man, as the King of the Jews; it must also critique the imagery of an omnipotent and omniscient God who heals spiritually while watching jealously over any human medical treatment or discovery in science. Instead, theology must trans-late what God's love means – and what the love of God means in view of suffering, to wit what God's compassion means (Haker 2017). Simone Weil has given us *one* way to understand that the experience of abandonment by God is not the result of a sadistic, un-empathic God. For John Caputo, a theology that leaves its ontotheological legacy behind, must begin with the understanding of the weakness of God (Caputo 2006).[28] God's weakness, I hold, is the ultimate, divine vulnerability: the openness of the divine lover for her beloved, the human being whom she has set free, to live the life of a natal and mortal being, in vulnerable agency, finite freedom,

---

28   I do not share Caputo's enthusiasm for the theology of the "event" but still think that he is
       right in insisting on the weakness of God.

and the capability to respond to the other, and, who knows, perhaps to the wholely Other (Celan 1978, 35f.).[29]

Bibliography

Anderson, Pamela Sue (2016): The transformative power of vulnerability. Online: http://enhancinglife.uchicago.edu/blog/the-transformative-power-of-vulnerability (last access 03/05/2019).

Bamberg, Michael (2006): Stories: Big or small: Why do we care? in: Narrative Inquiry 16:139-147.

Bamberg, Michael/Georkakopoulou, Alexandra (2008): Small stories as a new perspective in narrative and identity analysis, in: Text & Talk 28, 3: 377-396.

Benjamin, Jessica (1988): The bonds of love: psychoanalysis, feminism, and the problem of domination, vol. 1, New York: Pantheon Books.

Benjamin, Jessica (2017): Beyond doer and done to: recognition theory, intersubjectivity and the third, New York: Routledge.

Benjamin, Walter (1999): The Storyteller. Observations on the works of Nikolai Leskov (orig. 1936), in: Illuminations, edited by Hannah Arendt, 83-107. London: Pimlico.

Bernstein, J. M. (2011): Trust. On the real but almost always unnoticed, ever-changing foundation of ethical life, in: Metaphilosophy 42, 4: 395-416. Online: https://doi.org/10.1111/j.1467-9973.2011.01709.x (last access 03/08/2019).

Bernstein, J. M. (2015): Torture and dignity. An essay on moral injury, Chicago/London: The University of Chicago Press.

Bishop, Jeffrey P. (2011): The anticipatory corpse. Medicine, power, and the care of dying. Notre Dame studies in medical ethics, Notre Dame: Notre Dame Publisher.

Bleakley, Alan (2015): Medical humanities and medical education. How the medical humanities can shape better doctors, London/New York: Routledge, Taylor & Francis Group.

Blumenberg, Hans (2006): Beschreibung des Menschen, Frankfurt: Suhrkamp.

Bobbert, Monika (2000): Die Problematik des Krankheitsbegriffs und der Entwurf eines moralisch-normativen Krankheitsbegriffs im Anschluß an die Moralphilosophie von Alan Gewirth, in: Ethica 8, 4: 405-440.

Boorse, Christopher (2014): A second rebuttal on health, in: The journal of medicine and philosophy 39, 6: 683. Online: https://doi.org/10.1093/jmp/jhu035 (last access 03/08/2019).

---

29   Celan says that the poem, while speaking "in its own, its own, individual cause", is expected to speak *in the cause of an Other* – who knows, perhaps in the cause of the wholely Other" (emphasis there).

Caputo, John D. (2006): The weakness of God. A theology of the event, Bloomington: Indiana University Press.

Carel, Havi (2016): Phenomenology of illness. Oxford: Oxford University Press.

Cassell, Eric J. (2004): The nature of suffering and the goals of medicine, vol. 2., New York; Oxford: Oxford University Press.

Celan, Paul (1978): The Meridian (translated by Jerry Glenn), in: Chicago Review 29, 3: 29-40. Online: https://www.jstor.org/stable/25303702?seq=12#metadata_info_tab_ contents (last access 03/14/2019).

Dussel, Enrique (2014): Hermeneutics and critique from a liberation ethics perspective, in: Labyrinth. An international journal for philosophy 16, 1: 27-51. Online: http://dx.doi.org/10.25180/lj.v16i1.28 (last access 03/08/2019).

Flanagan, Tara (2017): Narrative medicine and health care ethics: Religious and literary approaches to patient identity and clinical practice. Dissertation: Loyola University Chicago.

Foucault, Michel (1978): The history of sexuality, vol. 1-3, London: Random House.

Foucault, Michel (2007): Security, territory, population. Lectures at the Collège de France, 1977-78, Basingstoke/New York: Palgrave Macmillan.

Frank, Arthur W. (1995): The wounded storyteller. Body, illness and the human condition, Chicago: University of Chicago Press.

Friend, Tad (2017): Silicon Valley's quest to live forever. Can billions of dollars' worth of high-tech research succeed in making death optional?, in: New Yorker 04/03/2017.

Gadamer, Hans-G. (1975): Truth and method, London: Sheed & Ward.

Gadamer, Hans-G. (1996): The enigma of health (orig. Über die Verborgenheit der Gesundheit, 1993). Stanford: Stanford University Press.

Gilson, Erinn C. (2014): The ethics of vulnerability. a feminist analysis of social life and practice, vol. 1, New York: Routledge.

Haker, Hille (1999): Moralische Identität. Literarische Lebensgeschichten als Medium ethischer Reflexion. Mit einer Interpretation der "Jahrestage" von Uwe Johnson, Tübingen: Francke.

Haker, Hille (2005): The fragility of the moral self, in: Harvard Theological Review 97, 4: 359-382.

Haker, Hille (2010): Narrative Ethik, in: Zeitschrift für Didaktik der Philosophie und Ethik 2: 74-83.

Haker, Hille (2015a): Ethik und Empirie, in: W. Schaupp (Ed.), Ethik und Empirie. Gegenwärtige Herausforderungen für Moraltheologie und Sozialethik. Freiburg i.Br.: Herder, 19-40.

Haker, Hille (2015b): Verletzlichkeit als Kategorie der Ethik, in: M. Bobbert (Ed.), Zwischen Parteilichkeit und Ethik. Schnittstellen von Klinikseelsorge und Medizinethik. Berlin/Münster: Lit, 195-225.

Haker, Hille (2016): Beyond the anticipatory corpse. Future perspectives for Bioethics, in: Journal of medicine and philosophy 41: 597-620.

Haker, Hille (2017): Compassion for justice, in: Concilium 2017, 4: 54-64.

Haker, Hille. (2019): Vulnerable agency. A conceptual and contextual analysis, in: J. Rothschild/M. Petrusek (Eds.), Dignity and conflict. Contemporary interfaith dialogue on the value and vulnerability of human life, Notre Dame: Notre Dame University Press.

Hercz, Gavril/Novak, Marta (2013): The challenges presented by the non-compliant patient, in: CANNT journal. Journal ACITN 23, 4: 30.

Kalish, Naomi (2012): Evidence-based spiritual care. A literature review, in: Current opinion in supportive and palliative care 6, 2: 242-246. Online: doi:10.1097/SPC.0b013e328353811c (last access 03/14/2019).

Kittay, Eva Feder (2016): A theory of justice as fair terms of social life given our inevitable dependency and our inextricable interdependency, in: D. Engster/M. Hamington (Eds.) Care ethics and political theory, Oxford Scholarship Online: Oxford University Press, 1-29.

Levinas, Emmanuel (1969): Totality and infinity. An essay on exteriority, Pittsburgh: Duquesne University Press.

Levinas, Emmanuel (1987): Time and the other and additional essays, Pittsburgh: Duquesne University Press.

Levinas, Emmanuel (1998): Otherwise than being, or beyond essence. Pittsburgh: Duquesne University Press.

Levinas, Emmanuel (2000): God, death, and time. Stanford, Calif.: Stanford University Press.

Lindemann Nelson, Hilde (2001): Damaged identities, narrative repair, Ithaca: Cornell University Press.

MacIntyre, Alasdair (1999): Dependent rational animals, Chicago: open court.

Merry, Michael (2004): On evil, sin, and suffering. Toward a hermeneutic of their relation, in: Journal of Pastoral Care & Counseling 58, 1-2: 75-82. Online: https://doi.org/10.1177/154230500405800109 (last access 03/08/2019).

Mieth, Dietmar (2002): Sozialethik als hermeneutische Ethik, in: Jahrbuch für Christliche Sozialwissenschaften 43: 217-240.

Nussbaum, Martha C. (2001): Upheavals of thought. The intelligence of emotions, Cambridge; New York: Cambridge University Press.

Parker, Jan/Bowman, Deborah/Kokanović, Renata (2018): Stories, narratives, scenarios in Medicine, in: Arts and humanities in higher education 17, 1: 3-19. Online: https://doi.org/10.1177/1474022217740300 (last access 03/08/2019).

Ricœur, Paul (1998): Critique and conviction. Conversations with François Azouvi and Marc de Launay. New York: Columbia University Press.

Ricœur, Paul (2005): The course of recognition, Cambridge, Mass.: Harvard University Press.

Rieff, David (2008): Swimming in a sea of death. A son's memoir, kindle ed. New York: Simon and Schuster.

Svenaeus, Fredrik (2014): The phenomenology of suffering in medicine and bioethics, in: Philosophy of medical research and practice 35, 6: 407-420. https://doi.org/10.1007/s11017-014-9315-3 (last access 03/08/2019).

Svenaeus, Fredrik (2015): The phenomenology of chronic pain. Embodiment and alienation, in: Continental philosophy review 48, 2: 107-122. Online: https://doi.org/10.1007/s11007-015-9325-5 (last access 03/08/2019).

Taylor, Charles (2016): The language animal. The full shape of the human linguistic capacity, Cambridge/Mass.: The Belknap Press of Harvard University Press.

Theunissen, Michael (1984): The other. Studies in the social ontology of Husserl, Heidegger, Sartre, and Buber (orig.: Der Andere: Studien zur Sozialontologie der Gegenwart, 1977). Cambridge MA: MIT Press.

Toombs, S. Kay (1992): The meaning of illness. A phenomenological account of the different perspectives of physician and patient, Dordrecht; Boston: Kluwer Academic Publishers.

Vetlesen, Arne J. (2004): A philosophy of pain, London: Reaktion books.

Waldenfels, Bernhard (2002): Bruchlinien der Erfahrung. Phänomenologie, Psychoanalyse, Phänomenotechnik, Frankfurt am Main: Suhrkamp.

Waldenfels, Bernhard (2008): The role of the lived-body in feeling, in: Continental philosophy review 41, 2: 127-142. Online: https://doi.org/10.1007/s11007-008-9077-6 (last access 03/08/2019).

Weil, Simone (1977): The love of God and affliction, in: George A. Panichas (Ed.), The Simone Weil Reader. New York: McKay, 439-468.

Zahavi, Dan (2014a): Empathy and other-directed intentionality, in: An international review of philosophy 33, 1: 129-142. Online: https://doi.org/10.1007/s11245-013-9197-4 (last access 03/08/2019).

Zahavi, Dan (2014b): Self and other. Exploring subjectivity, empathy, and shame. Oxford: Oxford University Press.

Medical Technology and the Body

Narrative Ethics in Simone de Beauvoir's A Very Easy Death

Tara Flanagan

Using narrative medicine as an interpretive framework, this chapter analyzes Simone de Beauvoir's account of her mother's final days in *A Very Easy Death* as representative of the social and experiential motivations for and consequences of using life-prolonging technology for dying patients. I place particular focus on medical aesthetics and how the event of death is shaped by the presence of medical technology both in the context of the hospital and in the hospice model of care. Surrounding a dying person in medical machinery creates a barrier that isolates a dying patient during a time when the physical presence of others can offer needed comfort. On the other hand, the presence of medical technology may provide benefits when considering the perspective of family members. The sight of medical equipment surrounding a patient's body assures those present that concrete efforts are being taken to preserve the life of a loved one. Also, the equipment used provides a therapeutic barrier from the physical reality of the dying process and the finality of death. This is not to say that medical technology should be used for these reasons, but that it can be beneficial for clinicians to understand family member's motivations when asking for extreme life-prolonging measures for patients at the end-of-life.

In *A Very Easy Death*, both family members, Mme de Beauvoir's daughters Simone and Poupette, recognize the futility of medical interventions in their mother's final days:

> "But what's the good of tormenting her, if she is dying? Let her die in peace", said Poupette, in tears...Dr N passed by me; I stopped him. White coat, white cap: a young man with an unresponsive face. "Why this tube? Why torture Maman, since there is no hope?" He gave me a withering look. "I am doing what has to be done" ... In the corridor he said "At dawn she scarcely had four hours left. I have brought her back to life." I did not venture to ask him "For what?" (de Beauvoir, 27-28)

Simone de Beauvoir's autobiographical narrative provides a resource in narrative medicine for ethical analysis of the reasons why medical interventions should not be standard practice for patients facing the end of life. Even though use of such equipment seems to provide some benefit for family members in materially demonstrating active care for their loved ones and distancing them from the prospect of death, ultimately the use of medical technology,

© BRILL SCHÖNINGH, 2022 | DOI:10.30965/9783657715428_011

and interventions such as surgery for patients at the end-of-life, can lead to distress for patients and family members alike. In lieu of equipment and interventions, frank talk about what to expect in the dying process is what best prepares patients and family members for the inevitable event of death. Such candor may be uncomfortable for clinicians unused to discussing the limits of medical care, but enduring this discomfort and having difficult conversations acknowledging the reality of death and what to expect in the dying process can provide patients and family members with the comfort they are seeking, displaced through requests for intervention.

De Beauvoir's narrative identifies reasons why clinicians should not relent to pressure from family members to use superfluous medical treatments at the end-of-life—primarily because, though initially such use might assuage the anxiety of patients and family members, ultimately such interventions can cause preventable and unnecessary pain. Honest talk about what to expect when facing death, such as that provided by clinicians in hospice and palliative care, can lessen the existential anxiety that precipitates the use of medical technology and interventions at life's end. A first-person narrative, de Beauvoir's *A Very Easy Death* illustrates the aesthetics and the experiential dimension of the use of medical technology for end-of-life patients from a family member's perspective. Offering autobiographical insight on the clinical experience, *A Very Easy Death* serves as a resource for moral reflection for those practicing methods in narrative medicine, particularly those who are interested in the phenomenological experience of the clinical encounter and ethical perspectives on clinical care.

Narrative medicine is an approach to medical care that seeks to deepen a clinician's ability to listen and respond to patients during the clinical encounter. Rita Charon, physician and literature scholar, developed narrative medicine as a framework for physicians, one in which they supplement their medical knowledge as practitioners with the interpersonal communication skills involved in engaging with patients. Methods in narrative medicine include close reading, reflective writing, interpretation of texts such as literature, and parallel charting (Charon 2008). Practitioners trained in narrative medicine frequently use fiction as source for clinical and personal reflection. In this chapter, I propose that autobiographical illness accounts from the family's perspective offer needed insight on the clinical experience. By reading and reflecting on the accounts provided by family members, clinicians can consider the clinical experience and its effects from the perspective of those who have lived through the experience, many of whom offer ethical insights on how care can be provided.

Hille Haker's scholarship on narrative medical ethics demonstrates that narrative bioethics approaches literature as offering both commentary and critique – commentary on the substance of the text and critique of the medical model as it is experienced by the patient (Haker 2006). Demonstrating the ways in which narrative bioethics is also literary hermeneutical bioethics, she says:

> Literary ethics directs the reader's attention to ethical questions posed in and by means of a literary text. It analyses them, in that it attempts to understand ethical questions as a function of the text, but above all it holds up the narrated and evoked world of the work in contrast to the existential and practical reality to which the ethical judgements and perspectives refer. (Ibid., 356)

Here, Haker speaks to the enterprise of narrative bioethics as one offering both critique and commentary when turning to literature as a source for moral reflection. Building on this, I believe that autobiographical illness accounts, such as the first-person perspective offered by Simone de Beauvoir, portrays both commentary and critique in and of itself. De Beauvoir is essentially engaging in the hermeneutical enterprise of narrative bioethics in her text, though she reverses the posture of the figure providing commentary. In narrative medicine, the clinician offers commentary on the ways in which works of art apply to the practice of medicine. In *A Very Easy Death*, de Beauvoir presents her commentary on the medicalized death of her mother, providing a critique of the medical model as experienced by family members involved in the clinical encounter. De Beauvoir's narrative models Haker's view of "literature as a medium *of* ethical reflection and *for* ethical reflection (Ibid., 358).

Clinical ethicists offer needed insight on how care is best provided in a way that honors a patient's dignity and autonomy. The perspective of family members, as they have experienced the fallout of depersonalized medicine firsthand, can supplement ethical analyses of clinical care and provide material for improving the clinical experience. Such first-person accounts provide resources for reflection for those studying narrative medicine, particularly for those interested in narrative medical ethics. By reading these narratives, clinicians can identify experiences of pain and suffering related to clinical care, thereby learning how to provide better care in the future. In *A Very Easy Death*, de Beauvoir describes her emotional response to witnessing the terminal decline of her mother and the care her mother receives in the hospital. By reading her account of her mother's death, clinicians can reflect on how patients and family members experience medical care at the end of life to supplement and expand their perspectives as care providers, taking time to question and examine their norms of care. In the commentary and critique I present here,

I examine de Beauvoir's account as a resource for considering reasons why family members request the use of life prolonging medical technology when their family members are terminal, even actively dying. Clinicians are often conflicted when faced with such requests (Kasman 2004), and narratives such as de Beauvoir's offer insight from the family's perspective on what motivates requests for highly technologized care for dying patients.

Examining the Use of Medical Technology at the End of Life

Questions about the appropriate use of medical technology often center on its use at the beginning of life, including ethical concerns regarding the just use of biotechnology with regard to cloning, stem cells, and other modalities of reproduction. A less glamorous application of technology is to end of life patients, particularly those facing imminent death in acute care units such as the ICU. Considering the pace of technological innovation and the growth of the aging demographic, the following question calls for reflection: What is the future of human death in a medical landscape marked by the use of medical technology? Medical technology, including resources such as defibrillators, feeding tubes, ventilators and even oxygen tanks, certainly has the power to save lives. For instance, for those with a chronic disease such as kidney failure, dialysis machines sustain their ability to live day-to-day. For those at the end of life, however, particularly patients with terminal diseases who are hospice eligible, technology is less oriented toward recovery and more oriented toward delaying death, creating the impression that a patient's life can continue on despite a terminal prognosis.

A study supported by the Robert Wood Johnson Foundation on care for the dying noted that half of the deaths in the United States happen in clinical settings, in which patients are "surrounded by the technologies of medicine, embedded in a highly specialized, sophisticated setting."[1] Many patients state that they would prefer to die at home; however, a consensus statement from the American College of Critical Care Medicine found that 22% of deaths in the United States occur in intensive care units – a highly technologized environment, where visiting hours are strictly limited (Truog et al. 2009, 953). Though a hospital setting offers continuous care for a patient as a patient approaches the end of life, the setting is one that is oriented toward curative, professional, technological care (Wenham/Pittard, 2009).

---

1   For a discussion of this 4-year study on preferences for end-of-life treatment, see Cahill 2005, 70f.

For terminal patients, for whom curative care can be considered futile, medical technology can be used for more than medical treatment; there are deeper reasons for the use of medical technology at the end of life, moving beyond its clinical function. Some overtreatment may be done at the family's request (Luce 2010), while at other times medical technology can be used to mask the reality of death as an unsettling biological event. The equipment can serve to camouflage the physical reality of death, figuratively and literally hiding the full reality of the dying body from sight. Instead of a visitor observing the dying body of another, the visitor sees tubes, plastic, metal, and other barriers. The medicalized death becomes a technologized event, insulated from any visceral human encounter.

The unnecessary use of medical technology for patients at the end-of-life occurs for a variety of reasons. Bioethicist Daniel Callahan (1993) suggests that there is a technological imperative when it comes to the use of medical equipment: that any device that can be used will be used, regardless of efficacy or need, merely because it exists as an option. Alternatively, a desire to avoid frank death-talk may fuel the use of medical technology; instead of discussing the unpleasant reality that a patient's condition is terminal, doctors and families alike may grasp at hope that equipment can be used to save or sustain a dying person. Finally, the use of medical technology may function as a therapeutic barrier, the machinery shielding or distracting the patient's family from the patient's declining body and creating the impression that the patient's condition is manageable.

In *A Very Easy Death*, Simone de Beauvoir's description of her mother's death illustrates the third of these points, bringing the aesthetics of death into sharp relief by describing how medical technology functions phenomenologically for dying patients, their clinical caregivers, and their visitors. In so doing, De Beauvoir's account of her mother's physical decline and diminishing autonomy reveals the extent to which de Beauvoir absorbs social expectations about what it means to be normatively embodied: to be in control, to be dignified, and to be in full health. De Beauvoir is disquieted by her formerly authoritative mother taking on a passive role, relinquishing control over her body, her relationships, and her environment. She recoils at the sight of her mother's wasting body and describes the hospital as a chaotic and degrading environment, one in which her mother's frail body is exposed to others in a manner that causes needless discomfort for both her mother and herself.

Family members in De Beauvoir's position may prefer a technologized environment such as that provided in the ICU. While the paradigmatic end-of-life scenario involves a research-obsessed physician pushing aggressive care onto vulnerable patients, it may as often be the family's desire that the patient die in an aesthetically managed way; this desire then driving the overuse of medical technology. The use of medical machinery at the end of life can serve a quasi-therapeutic function in that it cushions family members from immediacy of the dying human body, and ultimately from the reality that we cannot over-power death.[2]

A Very Easy Death as Narrative Case Study

Simone de Beauvoir's account of her mother's final days in *A Very Easy Death* (1985) addresses the alterity of the dying body, the limits of autonomy and the necessity of care, and the symbolic, social, and aesthetic functions of medi-cal technology for patients at the end of life. De Beauvoir offers a daughter's perspective on the death of her mother, and describes the ways the experience shaped her perspective on medical care at the end of life. In addition to the grief she feels over the loss of her parent, her mother's death serves as a har-binger of her own; facing the decline of her mother's body means facing the impending decline of her body, the loss of her agency, and the end of her life. Her mother's frail, dying body in front of her, previously a resilient, life-giving body, stands as a stark reminder of her own mortality. De Beauvoir speaks to this connection when she describes her mother's funeral as being a dress rehearsal for her own. In her narrative, De Beauvoir describes the struggle her mother had letting go of agency and transitioning from a self-sufficient life on her own to that of a patient in the hospital, dependent on others in a space that she could not control. Her mother ultimately relents her hold on personal agency and accepts her new role as a dependent patient; one could say she demonstrates a passive form of agency here – choosing to receive care from others.[3] However, her daughter remained uncomfortable with her mother's relational transition and physical decline.

Madame de Beauvoir, age 78, falls while at home and is admitted to a hos-pital to treat a broken femur. While admitted, the physicians discover intes-tinal blockage and she is diagnosed with cancer. Though lucid for most of her stay, her diagnosis is withheld from her, and the clinicians maintain that rather than having cancer – one of her great fears in life according to her daughter – she instead has peritonitis and she believes, due in no small part

---

2   Daniel Callahan offers an economic analysis of the use of medical technology (Callahan 2009) This article primarily attends to the experiential costs (and gains).

3   See Haker 2004. In this article Haker, draws on Emmanuel Levinas' text (Levinas 2000) and Jacques Derrida (Derrida 1999) to show how resisting care can function as a form of agency One could say that the ability to receive care as well as resist care is a form of agency as well.

to the deceit of her caregivers, that she will recover. She stays thirty days in the hospital, attended to by medical staff and visited by her daughters, Simone and Poupette, until she dies. Her death, witnessed by Poupette, was a struggle, not the "very easy death" the nurse describes afterward (Beauvoir 1985, 88). De Beauvoir's account of her mother's death discloses the experiential aspects of the turn toward death, particularly the ways in which an institutional context shapes care, with special attention to the aesthetics, including the grotesque features, of a dying body embedded in medical equipment.

Additionally, *A Very Easy Death* describes the challenges involved when individuals who value autonomy are forced to transition, due to illness or increasing frailty, to relying on assistance from others to engage in activities of daily life. Madame de Beauvoir had been living independently in an apartment when she had her fall. Used to caring for herself, and before that caring for her daughters and husband, once she became hospitalized it was difficult for her to receive care. The nurse described her as seeming "so ashamed of being a nuisance," though ultimately she did end up relaxing into the experience of being cared for and attended to by the nursing staff (12; 23). In contrast to her mother's eventual embrace of her status as recipient of care rather than as care-provider, her daughter is challenged by the bodily dependence of her mother, seeing dependence as a form of lifelessness, calling her mother's body a "poor defenseless carcass turned and manipulated by professional hands" (Ibid., 21). In addition to noting the impersonal, objectifying treatment of her mother by the clinical staff, she views the body needing care as a corpse-body. Her mother's weakening, dependent body exposed the truth about the decline and upcoming death of her mother.

De Beauvoir is moved to disgust by the sight of her mother's diminishment and reflects back to the memory of her mother in her vitality. The physical decline of her mother, and her mother's relinquishment of agency, unsettles her; she grieves the loss of her strong, independent, healthy mother. She recoils from the sight of her mother's body, with its smell and creaturely weakness. For others, the buffer created by a technological barrier may be a welcome one, protecting the viewer from that which is unpleasant to see, smell, and hear – the dying body, the sour odor of sickness, the gasps of air hunger. Rather than the ICU offering a dystopian context for end of life care, it can instead provide a welcome respite from the realities of death, offering a tidy, efficient, highly managed space, an environment in which the repellent features of the dying body are hidden from sight. Her response to her mother's body is one of deep discomfort, discomfort with the exposed body, with surrendered agency, and with what she perceives to be undignified medical care. The sources of her uneasiness point to her preference for the normative, healthy body, one that is in control, independent, and fully agential. The clinical move to cover the body, then, does not necessarily mean that clinicians are detached, impersonal scientists who do not care for the patient as person; rather the move to cover the body with medical equipment, in contexts such as the ICU, can be the preference of the patient's family rather than the result of a single-minded desire to aggressively treat patients on the part of clinicians.

Regarding the topic of agency and her mother's increasing need for care-giving, de Beauvoir comes to recognize that she had a concretized view of her mother that did not include her mother as a dependent creature. Seeing her mother in bed had, "wrenched her out of the framework, the role, the set of images in which I had imprisoned her" (Ibid., 20). In addition to being unsettled by her mother's frail body, she, like her mother, was uneasy with the idea of her mother as a recipient of care rather than a provider of care. Her view of her mother was disrupted by the woman she saw on the hospital bed in front of her, but this disruption forced her to examine the multiple dimensions of her mother's personhood. She realizes that her mother was in fact many different mothers – her beloved mother when de Beauvoir was a child, an oppressive mother when she was a teenager, and now an old mother, dying (Ibid., 103). She also acknowledges that her mother had a life outside of her parenting role that is opaque to her.

Her account reveals the discomfort that can come when one faces the social and material breakdown of the human body in the turn toward death – the shifts in roles and relationships and the limits of agency, including the limits of one's control of the body. De Beauvoir's memory of her mother is of a woman poised and in control of her environment. De Beauvoir interprets her mother's experience in the hospital as impersonal and undignified. In the hospital, her mother becomes a body, a "carcass", connoting that she is treated as dead already. Rather than moving freely and being in control of her body, she is handled by the staff in a detached, even brusque, manner almost as if she were an object. Her body is not properly covered, exposing her nakedness to strangers in what her daughter interprets to be a degrading manner. Though her mother appeared to experience no distress at the display of her body (Ibid., 19), some may see this neglect of dignity as an ethical issue, naming these day-to-day experiences of hospital and nursing home residents the concerns of "everyday ethics" having to do with "indignities and losses of ordinary life" (Johnson 2005, 239). Daniel Sulmasy and Paul Ricœur similarly speak about the accumulation of small indignities that patients experience in the hospital (Sulmasy 2009; Ricœur 2000).

However, is her mother's experience undignified or is de Beauvoir uncomfortable with facing the direct reality of her mother's declining body in front of her? Her discomfort with the reality of her mother's death can be one of the reasons behind her motivation to cover her mother's body. One can locate in the ICU the extreme form of this desire to conceal the body in a technological cover, one that veils both the ugliness of the sick body and creates a gauzy distance from the disturbing event of death. Though Callahan argues that the very existence of technology leads to its use, I add that it is the combination of discomfort with the dying body, such as that described by de Beauvoir, combined with the option of a technologized death that propels the use of medical machinery for dying patients. There is an impulse to cover the exposed body with a gown or a bed cover; in the ICU this impulse is radicalized through the use of medical technology.

De Beauvoir notes the struggle she had visiting her mother in the hospital and encountering her transfigured physical presence there, a presence she admits she would rather not see. Her mother also expressed awareness that her body had changed, particularly after she had a stroke while in the hospital, saying, "I had a feeling my eyes were in the middle of my cheeks, and that my nose was [...] bent. It's odd" (Beauvoir 1985, 59). Her description of her face can be seen as representative of one's uncanny relationship with one's body at the end of life. Simone accepts the reality of her mother's impending death but grieves her mother's physical changes and diminishment.

Medical equipment such as that used in acute care contexts, can create a false sense of life: the heart still beats, the chest still rises and falls, skin is still warm. In such a context, clinicians and family members can maintain the comforting illusion of control over death because they control the use of the medical equipment. Because death often occurs in clinical contexts such as the ICU, with its dominating presence of medical technology that shields the visitor from the reality of death, the tension between the presence of equipment and the presence of those accompanying patients who are dying in such a context calls for close attention. Narratives such as de Beauvoir's serve as a resource for discussion and ethical reflection for clinicians reflecting on practices of care at the end-of-life.

The Turn toward Medicalized Death

How did death come to be seen as a reality that cannot be faced directly, but one that has to be covered up in the accouterments of the modern hospital? Callahan, bioethicist and cofounder of the Hastings Center, analyzes the development of how death in the United States came to be framed as an event that can be managed and controlled in medical institutions. In his article, "Frustrated Mastery: The Cultural Context of Death in America" (Callahan

1995), Callahan shows how the concept of a death-as-foe shapes how dying persons are treated, lifting up the correlation that exists between the medical and social concept of death and the experience of death. He describes the ways cultural understandings of death influence how an individual prepares for and interprets the event of death, be it the event of one's own future death or the death of another person. When death is conceived as adversarial, simply one more disease to be overcome, this biological, inevitable event in every human's life comes to be seen as a failure of medicine, even a personal failure on the part of the patient. Death becomes an embarrassment, a disruption, something that was not supposed to happen, something to fight, resist or conquer. As such, it is understandable that the aggressive use of intrusive technology to prolong life would be seen as both expected and beneficial (Callahan 2003).

In addition to the dramatic financial costs of the current use of medical technology to prolong life and delay death, there is another cost: the loss of the experience of death as an intimate event, as a moment, not of failure, but as a deeply personal event, the final moment of an irreplaceable person's life (Sulmasy 2009; 2006). Callahan speaks to this loss when he talks about the "impersonality, even unwitting cruelty, of death in a technologic cocoon" (Callahan 1995, 228). In addition to the loss of the time of death as a sacred, if solemn, event, there is another loss as well, that of a witness, of another person to provide presence with the one dying. Medical technology can, in a sense, be seen as a sort of proxy, a proxy that, if one is dying in a hospital, renders the presence of the medical professional at the time of death unnecessary. It is important to note here, that in addition to dying in pain, one of the great fears people have about death is the possibility of dying alone (Lynn/Teno 1997). Ultimately, equipment cannot replace the role of a person there to be present with a patient as he or she experiences death. Regarding the use of medical technology as a form of proxy, the claim here is not that clinicians intentionally abandon patients, but that medical technologies can function as a form of physical presence with a patient, though an insufficient one.

Recent scholarship on medical epistemology demonstrates how aesthetics, specifically how death is viewed in the hospital, affects patient care. Jeffrey Bishop uses the term "palliating gaze," supplementing Foucault's term "medical gaze," to describe how palliative care perceives the body as one that can be managed medically as it progresses toward the event of death (Bishop 2011; Foucault 1994). Bishop notes that how dying patients are regarded changed over time, the holistic view of the person in the original model of hospice care as established by Cicely Saunders morphing into the totalizing view of palliative care as an arm of the hospital system. Callahan, though he similarly inveighs against the impersonal nature of clinical care for terminal patients, offers hope that medical culture can change. By showing that interpretations of death are historical constructs, Callahan in turn lifts up the possibility that the cultural atmosphere around the event of death can be modified, ideally restructured to frame death as natural event. Hospice physician Ira Byock (1998) confirms Callahan's position on the historical nature of death as a medical event in "Living and Dying with Medical Technology," noting that how death is viewed shapes how the dying are treated, or, with the use of medical technology, over-treated. Byock calls for a new vision for how death is understood in contemporary U.S. culture, not as something we are to fight as though it could be conquered or hidden through the use of medical technology, but as a biological, and for some spiritual or religious, event that does not require such strenuous resistance. What is missing in the medical understanding of death as an adversary, or, to use the aggressive, militaristic language that is often used, as a "battle to be won" (Sontag 1979), is honesty about the limits of human power and recognition of the finitude of human life. The reductionist understanding of death as a medical event that happens to our bodies also ignores facets of our humanity that include our bodies but extend beyond them, our need for touch, for instance, and our existence as religious and social creatures.

Also turning to medical epistemology, Lisa Cahill examines how cultural understandings of death in the United States shape how patients are treated (Cahill 2005, 71f.). She names three features of contemporary American thought that inform how death is viewed: 1) the privileged position given to an individualism centered on autonomy and self-determination, 2) the medicalization of social problems, and 3) the refusal to accept that life has limits. She reframes this paradigm to include an awareness of humans as relational, meaning-oriented beings that do not have complete control over how the world functions. Aligning with Callahan, her work shows that how death is interpreted correlates directly with medical standards of care for dying patients. If the primary goal is to keep a person alive, all means possible to make this happen will be considered part of the plan of care, regardless of the cost, and without recognizing that a lingering, medicalized, institutionalized death may be against the wishes of many patients. By reframing how death is understood, she hopes to foster an acceptance of medical limits and improve the quality of care for patients at the end of life.

Medical Epistemology in the Hospice Model of Care

Hospice offers an alternative experience of death, in which clinicians such as nurses, social workers, and chaplains are candid about what to expect in the dying process, directly addressing the grotesque aspects of death and dying,

and potentially obviating the need for medical technology to shield one from
the discomfort that can arise from encountering a dying patient. The model
is not anti-technology; hospice orders often include the use of minor medical
equipment such as oxygen, walkers, and a hospital bed. However, when medical equipment is used in a home or living facility, it functions differently than
it does in the hospital. In the hospital, the oxygen tube represents the larger
medical apparatus involved in, to use Bishop's language, managing death. In
contrast to how equipment functions medically and symbolically at the hospital, in home-based hospice care, or other contexts where medical technology
has a low profile, such equipment serves in what Callahan calls a functional
manner, assisting rather than dominating the body of the patient. Because
honesty about the dying process frames the philosophy of care for hospice
patients, the equipment used does not serve to hide or distract from the reality
of the patient's upcoming death.

Rather than offering a romanticized version of "natural" death, the hospice
model promotes educating the patient and family about what to expect in the
dying process, that skin may be cold or turn blue, that breath may become
labored or gurgly, that delusions may occur or a person may turn inward and
not care about family or major life events like birthdays or anniversaries. Death
in the hospice model is less managed than it is in the hospital, and possibly
more uncomfortable for the witnesses involved. However, forthright conversations about the dying process can prepare patients and families for what
to expect and in so doing can reduce the discomfort that comes from being
shocked by the sight of the vulnerable, declining body. In the narrative written
by Simone de Beauvoir, one of the reasons her mother's death was difficult
to witness was because the clinicians tried to soften the experience. Due to
this interpretive cushion, the patient and family were unprepared for what to
expect. Also, because her mother was never told her diagnosis, she was denied
the opportunity to interpret her death on her own. This is not to say that her
experience in the hospital would have been positive had she known she had
terminal cancer, only that the opportunity to encounter and consider the final
limit of her life was missed.

Though the hospice model of care exists as an option for terminal patients
now, when Simone de Beauvoir's mother died in 1963, it did not yet exist as an
established option for treatment.[4] Nevertheless, her death shows how medical

---

4 Cicely Saunders formally established the hospice model of care for terminal patients with
   the opening of St. Christopher's Hospice in London in 1967. The first hospice program in the
   United States, Connecticut Hospice, was established in 1974 by nurse Florence Wald, who
   had worked at St. Christopher's.

technology can function both clinically and aesthetically, shaping the experience of death as both a biological and a social event. When normative embodiment means physical flourishing, the impulse to cover or hide the sick and dying body is unsurprising. In hospice, the sick and dying body is recognized and named by clinicians, structuring the event of death so that it is not perceived as a medical or biological aberration. Hospice is not a utopian model for end-of-life medicine or the "hero" to the hospital "villain," a common, but too easy binary for distinguishing the two. Instead hospice is redefining death as natural, and bringing this life event back to the realm of ordinary human experience. Futile care is something we resort to out of our hope that we and those we love will not die. Therefore, we keep treating a terminal person and keep covering them in machinery to hide what we do not want to see. We need to go the other direction and accept the limits of our technical power, normalize death as shared life event, and raise up the benefits of human contact including physical presence with those who are dying.

Ultimately, the question we now face is how we want the future of human dying, and of our own deaths, to unfold. Is the benefit of technology in extending one's life and shrouding the reality of death worth the loss of this deeply personal, relational, even sacred, experience? Medical technology exists as a qualified good, and its physical and symbolic presence for patients at the end of life calls for careful attention to both its benefits as well as its costs. In contrast to the heroic, but ultimately vain, ambition of technologically invasive care for the terminally ill, hospice recognizes the reality of human frailty and in so doing frees the dying patient from the physical, emotional, and spiritual burden of intrusive care at the end of life. Furthermore, the overall role of medical technology is minimized in the hospice model of care, thereby increasing the possibility of direct human contact for the dying patient, through touch or even the mere physical presence of another person in the room, an option that is not always available in intensive care units.

De Beauvoir's account discloses the influence of a technology-based medical epistemology on the event of death, one shaped by the institutional context and the medical equipment used to heal, or hide, the dying body. Her narrative of her mother's death also demonstrates the role aesthetics plays with regard to the hospital as the site of death. A context dominated by medical technology can cloak the dying body such that a person loses identity and becomes an object, hiding the dying body from sight and maintaining the false comfort that a cure for one's predicament is possible. Alternatively, it can provide a cover or distraction from the unwelcome sight of the ill or dying body and the reality of the body's final limit. In Simone de Beauvoir's case, she demonstrates an impulse to cover her mother's body to conceal the weakness and fragility of a woman she looked up to in life as strong-willed and independent. Her mother's physical decline causes her to be uneasy, even disgusted – it is in situations such as hers that the managed care provided in the ICU may be perceived as providing a form of comfort through control of the appearance the dying body. Candor about what to expect in the dying process, provided to patients and family members receiving hospice care, can mitigate this need to cover the body.

Bibliography

Ariès, Philippe (1974): Western attitudes toward death. From the Middle Ages to the Present, Baltimore: Johns Hopkins University Press.

Ariès, Philippe (1981): The hour of our death, New York: Random House.

Beauvoir, Simone de (1985): A very easy death, New York: Pantheon.

Bishop, Jeffrey Paul (2011): The anticipatory corpse. Medicine, power, and the care of the dying, Notre Dame, Ind.: University of Notre Dame Press.

Byock, Ira (1998): Dying well. Peace and possibilities at the end of life, New York: Riverhead Books.

Cahill, Lisa Sowle (2005): Theological bioethics. Participation, justice, and change. Washington, D.C.: Georgetown University Press.

Callahan, Daniel (1993): The troubled dream of life. In search of peaceful death, New York: Simon & Schuster.

Callahan, Daniel (2003): Living and dying with medical technology, in: Critical care medicine 31, 5: 344-346.

Callahan, Daniel (2009): Taming the beloved beast. How medical technology costs are destroying our Health Care System, Princeton: Princeton University Press.

Charon, Rita (2008): Narrative medicine. Honoring the stories of illness, New York: Oxford University Press.

Derrida, Jacques (1999): Adieu to Emmanuel Levinas, Stanford, Californien: Stanford University Press.

Foucault, Michel (1994): The birth of the clinic. An archaeology of medical perception, New York: Vintage Books.

Haker, Hille (2004): The fragility of the moral self, in: Harvard theological review 97, 4: 359-381.

Haker, Hille (2006): Narrative bioethics, in: C. Rehmann-Sutter/M. Düwell/D. Mieth, (Eds.), Bioethics in cultural contexts. Reflections on methods and finitude, 353-376, Dordrecht: Springer.

Hoover, Donald, et al. (2002): Medical expenditures during the last year of life. Findings from the 1992-1996 Medicare current beneficiary survey, in: Health services research 37, 6: 1625-1642.

Johnson, S. (2005): Living and dying in nursing homes, in: K. Doka/B. Jennings/ C.A. Corr (Eds.), Ethical dilemmas at the end of life, Washington, D.C.: Hospice foundation of America.

Kasman, Deborah (2004): When is medical treatment futile? A guide for students, residents, and physicians, in: Journal of general internal medicine 19, 10: 1053-1056.

Levinas, Emmanuel (2000): God, death, and time, Stanford, Calif.: Stanford University Press.

Luce, John M. (2010): End-of-life decision making in the intensive care unit, in: American Journal of respiratory and critical care medicine 182, 1: 6-11.

Lynn, Joanne/Teno, Joan M. (1997): Perceptions by family members of the dying experience of older and seriously ill patients, in: Annals of internal medicine 126, 2: 97-106.

Pellegrino, Edmund D./Schulman, Adam/Merill, Thomas W. (2009): Human dignity and bioethics, Notre Dame, Ind: University of Notre Dame Press.

Ricœur, Paul (2000): Prudential judgment, deontological judgment and reflexive. Judgment in medical ethics, in: P. Kemp/J. Rendtorff/N. Mattsson Johansen, Bioethics and biolaw, vol. 1: Judgment of Life, Copenhagen: Rhodos.

Sontag, Susan (1979): Illness as metaphor, New York: Vintage Books.

Sulmasy, Daniel (2009): Spirituality, religion, and clinical care, in: Chest 135, 6: 1634-42.

Sulmasy, Daniel (2006): The rebirth of the clinic. An introduction to spirituality in health care, Washington, D.C.: Georgetown University Press.

Truog, Robert D., et al. (2008): Recommendations for end-of-life care in the intensive care unit. Consensus statement by the American College of Critical Care Medicine, in: Critical Care Medicine 36, 3: 953-963.

Wenham, Tim/Pittard, Alison (2009): Intensive care unit environment: Continuing education in anesthesia, in: Critical Care & Pain 9, 6: 178-83.

Prenatal Genetic Testing & the Complicated Quest for a Healthy Baby

Christian Ethics in Conversation with Genetic Counselors

Aana Marie Vigen

Introduction

I was thrilled to be pregnant. While I did not want to know the sex, I fervently hoped that it was a healthy baby. I was over 35 and that fact categorized me as "advanced maternal age" and thus deemed at higher than normal risk for having a baby with a congenital abnormality. But what kind of information did I want?

Prenatal genetics can give pregnant women and their loved ones *a lot* to think about. Yet, it is also possible to have genetic testing without giving it much thought or without being fully aware one is having it. Moreover, especially if one lives in poverty and/or is uninsured in the United States, it is quite possible to miss out on sufficient prenatal care, let alone be given options regarding genetic testing.

For my part, I did not want to over-medicalize my pregnancy; yet I wanted the expertise (and reassurance) of the latest advances in medicine. Simply put, like a good American consumer, I wanted everything! Moreover, given my socio-economic and racial identities as a white woman (PhD., fully-employed, ample medical insurance), I had long been socialized to expect that I could exercise my autonomy – that I had options and a strong say in what kind of medical care I would receive.

When I consider topics in bioethics, questions of inequality invariably shape how I think about them. After giving birth, I began to wonder about the perspectives of pregnant women with less generous medical insurance than me and/or with less social clout – education, language abilities, white skin color. I also wanted to know more about the world of genetic counselors, especially those who work with vulnerable populations. Over time, I framed my central question in this way: Given the U.S. context of ever-advancing and complex genetic technologies, a hallowed free market economy and mindset, and pernicious socio-economic, gender, and racial-ethnic inequities, what will help pregnant women and their loved ones – especially those marginalized by society's structures of power and privilege – navigate prenatal genetics with

© BRILL SCHÖNINGH, 2022 | DOI:10.30965/9783657715428_012

a robust sense of moral agency and how might Christian ethics contribute to this endeavor?

This question contrasts with a wearisome opposition that often frames both Christian reproductive ethics and public policy debates in which fault lines are drawn between human dignity and sanctity of fetal life vs. respect for women's choice and autonomy. I find the narrow emphasis on individual rights and autonomy – found in both pro-choice and pro-life constituencies as Catholic ethicist Lisa Sowle Cahill reveals – increasingly unsatisfying. Cahill puts the crux of the matter well as she explains the difference, which emphasizing solidarity, rather than individual rights, can make in broadening our collective moral vision:

> An ethos of solidarity is a contrast to the ethos of liberal individualism that currently pervades both the pro-choice and pro-life movements. The public advocacy of both focused on individual rights that clash irremediably with the right or needs of others ... Such debates serve merely as a distraction from the fact that 'liberal' society is in reality ordered so as to exclude from social viability many of those to whom full 'personhood' is granted in the abstract. (Cahill 2005, 180)

In other words, we fail greatly as a society when we brandish signs that proclaim a strong defense of fetal life/rights *or* of women's lives and rights to bodily integrity and self-determination, but do very little by way of laws and policies and tax codes that would provide concrete support for children and women in their daily lives.[1]

Moreover, this dichotomy between "life and choice" may not adequately address the concerns of women who most need reproductive care and information, or of the healthcare professionals who attend to them. Ultimately, I hope to make a modest and constructive intervention regarding how central questions in respect of prenatal genetics are framed.

Three general areas of analysis structure what follows: 1. A snapshot of U.S. prenatal genetics; 2. Insights from ethnographic interviews with genetic counselors in light of the larger U.S. social context; 3. Tentative connections to Christian norms. This chapter grows out of a larger research endeavor that includes additional ethnographic interviews with Black and/or Latina new moms and with OB-GYNs (obstetrician-gynecologist). While more theologians

---

1 "The clash between the 'rights of the unborn' and the 'rights of women' comes across as a zero-sum game, skewed by the tacit belief of many that women in poverty, especially if they are members of racial and ethnic minorities, do not deserve assistance ... Clearly, abortion cannot be addressed apart from large issues of social justice, issues that cannot be surfaced, much less resolved, on a liberal model of social relationships." (Cahill 2005, 180f.)

and ethicists have begun to incorporate qualitative research methods into their works, it still represents a growing edge in theology (Vigen 2006; Scharen/ Vigen 2011; Browning 2014). I contend that Christian ethics is enriched when scholars cultivate a contextual sense of the field and allow some of the normative categories to emerge through attentive listening to people immersed in the moral issues at stake. Theologically put, this approach makes the case that taking God's incarnation seriously necessarily means taking human experience seriously.

A Snapshot of U.S. Reproductive Genetics

A Note on Terminology

Designations such as "birth defects", "congenital abnormality", and "genetic disorder" may imply a value judgment. Some authors (Becker 2011; Dollar 2012) who identify with disability rights prefer terms such as "genetic condition". They rightly note that not all deviations from the norm disrupt functioning or flourishing.

I find both "genetic condition" and "congenital abnormality" to be useful and appropriate terms. "Abnormal" in a medical context is often used to indicate a problem in function of an organ or tissue, as in the case of an abnormal pap smear, mammogram, brain development, or cardiac valve. The U.S. Centers for Disease Control (CDC) discusses birth defects in this way:

> Birth defects are structural changes present at birth that can affect almost any part or parts of the body (e.g. heart, brain, foot). They may affect how the body looks, works, or both. Birth defects can vary from mild to severe. The well-being of each child affected with a birth defect depends mostly on which organ or body part is involved and how much it is affected. Depending on the severity of the defect and what body part is affected, the expected lifespan of a person with a birth defect may or may not be affected. (CDC 2018c)

Thus, I use the term "birth defects" to signify not only a difference or variation, but a problem in the structural functioning of a human organ or system. Again, this distinction is open to interpretation and debate, as many who are deaf and also those who identify as LGBTQIA rightfully make clear.

U.S. Live Birth & Infant Mortality Statistics

In 2015, out of nearly 4 million live births, over 23,000 infants died before their first birthday (CDC 2019). The US infant mortality rate is nearly twice as high as peer industrialized nations (Rettner 2014). Why do so many U.S. infants die in these early months? Per the CDC, birth defects, many with associated genetic markers, are a leading cause (CDC 2019), "accounting for 20% of all infant deaths" (Mathews et al. 2015, 9). Overall, of the roughly 4 million annual live births, approximately 120,000 will have a congenital abnormality. The March of Dimes adds: "There are thousands of different birth defects, affecting the structure or function of every part of the human body … Currently, about 70 percent of the causes of birth defects are unknown"[2].

U.S. Prenatal Screening & Testing Practices

ACOG considers genetic screening to be a part of routine prenatal care and recommends that all women – regardless of age – be offered it (ACOG/SMFM 2016) Thus, the majority of women – especially if they receive early prenatal care – will be offered at least basic screening, often via a first trimester blood test and ultrasound. It is possible that not all the reasons for this initial screening may be clearly spelled out to patients. Three of the genetic counselors with whom I spoke indicated significant experience with having patients in their office who did not understand that they were having genetic screening or what this screening means. They spoke of the anxiety and confusion that this can cause. Two of them commented that many OB/GYNS are not skilled in explaining or interpreting the screening results, especially if they return with any sign of abnormal result, much less the complex field of genetics.

In any event, for those women with an abnormal result and/or those deemed at higher than normal risk of having a genetic abnormality (e.g. age, history of inherited genetic condition, prior pregnancy with a genetic anomaly, diabetes, obesity, history of drug use, infection during pregnancy, exposure to toxins), ACOG recommends a follow up with a more invasive, diagnostic test (chorionic villus sampling – CVS or amniocentesis).[3] A key distinction is screening vs. diagnostic. The three genetic counselors all testified to abundant confusion

---

2 http://www.marchofdimes.com/research/birth-defects-research.aspx.

3 Sarah Morgan, a genetic counselor, explained:

    ACOG recommends that all women – regardless of age – be offered a first trimester screen as part of routine prenatal care. The ideal is for pregnant women to have the 1st trimester bun screen – a blood test and ultrasound – but you have to be between 11 weeks 3 days and 13 weeks 6 days, a rather limited window. If they miss that window then there is the Quad screen in the 2nd trimester (with or without an ultrasound, depending on the calculated gestational age). The Quad Screen has a higher false positive rate and a lower detection rate than the 1st trimester screen.

    She emphasized:

    50 percent of pregnancies are unplanned, so women do not know they are pregnant until the 11-13 week window. So, then they have the quad screen. For patients who are eligible for the cell-free screen, they can do as early as 10 weeks. There is not technically an end date for

on this point. The various *screening* tests, available in the first and second tri-mesters give statistical probabilities. In other words, they can tell if there is greater or less probability for a particular patient that a congenital condition may be present. For a definitive *diagnosis*, one must have either the CVS or amniocentesis.[4]

A relatively new screening option – "cell-free DNA" (cfDNA) – is quickly changing prenatal care protocols. It is non-invasive, can be done as early as 10 weeks in pregnancy and is very accurate (though not diagnostic). It is most commonly used in the U.S. to screen for sex, fetal rhesus (Rh) blood type, and Trisomy 21 (Down syndrome), 18, and 13 (Mayo Clinic 2018).[5] Presently, ACOG recommends it only to those at a higher than normal risk.[6] However, there are indications that its use is increasing significantly in some U.S. clinical contexts (e.g. Greenfieldboyce 2015). Much depends on what kind of medical insurance a pregnant woman has, and on what health providers are most accustomed to offering. It is relatively expensive and not always covered by insurance policies.

What Are We Testing For?

Prenatal genetic tests have been developed for over 800 genetic conditions (Brody 2013). In the future, it may be possible to test for thousands. Yet in 2018 in the U.S., barring cases with a particular family history for specific diseases such as Tay-Sachs or Cystic fibrosis, a relatively defined number of congenital abnormalities are the ones most routinely focused upon: Trisomy 13, 18, 21; sex chromosome abnormalities; Spina bifida and other neural tube defects such as Anencephaly; and various cardiovascular, gastrointestinal, and muscular-skeletal abnormalities (CDC 2018a). Several of these diagnoses often have associated genetic markers.

---

this test, but they like to do it before 20 weeks to allow time for informed decision making regarding the pregnancy – continue, terminat e.

Follow up phone conversation with Sarah Morgan, 1/6/14. See also ACOG's recommenda-tions, revised March 2016 (ACOG/SMFM 2016).

4   For more information: https://www.acog.org/Patients/FAQs/Prenatal-Genetic-Screening-Tests.

5   It may also be used to screen for increased risks of other select conditions such as Trisomy 16, 22; Prader-Willi syndrome, a missing or extra sex chromosome, etc.

6   A 2015 recommendation: "Given the performance of conventional screening methods, the limitations of cell-free DNA screening performance, and the limited data on cost-effectiveness in the low-risk obstetric population, conventional screening method remain the most appropriate choice for first-line screening for most women in the general obstetric population" (ACOG/SMFM 2015, 5. Online: https://s3.amazonaws.com/cdn.smfm.org/pub-lications/198/download-5bae59126b5983e1f41757b0a9c8db0c.pdf).

Down syndrome is the most common chromosomal abnormality, occurring in one out of 691 births per year (Ibid.). Spina bifida is also fairly common. All three genetic counselors emphasized the wide range in severity in both diagnoses and in how much no one can know about the specific abilities or problems a particular baby born with either condition will have.

Moreover, while some congenital disorders are clearly caused by one factor, others are caused by a complex mix or an unknown cause. The CDC explains:

> For most birth defects, we think they are caused by a complex mix of factors. These factors include our genes (information inherited from our parents), our behaviors, and things in the environment. But, we don't fully understand how these factors might work together to cause birth defects. (CDC 2018c)

Thus, genetic anomalies constitute one important piece of a larger, complex puzzle.

For some women, genetic family histories constitute a particularly significant part of their health profile – e.g. women who suffer from or who have biological family member(s) with diseases that are known to be directly linked to genetic factors. Some individuals with such family histories want to learn a lot about their genetic profiles during pregnancy while others want less or no information. Similarly, some want to know the sex and others do not. Genetic testing can be – and is – used for sex selection purposes.[7] However, ultrasound technology by itself is picking up this information earlier and earlier. Two of the genetic counselors noted being asked on occasion by prenatal patients about sex selection, but that this was not overly common. Both noted the general consensus among both the professions of genetic counseling and OB/GYNS in the U.S. against using prenatal genetic information for sex selection purposes.

In a related matter, I learned from the genetic counselors that they do *not* generally prenatally screen for adult onset diseases – breast cancer genetic markers, Huntington's disease, Alzheimer's – and that this practice too is generally frowned upon by prenatal health professionals. Dory told me that in her 17 years of experience, no prenatal patient has asked her to do an adult onset test. Similarly, all three reported that within their prenatal contexts, patients are not asking for genetic tests to determine if their child will have blue eyes, be a stellar athlete, have perfect pitch, or be gay. While these requests may be made elsewhere, these particular counselors do not see this as preoccupation or interest in their particular patient populations.

---

7   The eager consumer can buy an over the counter gender test that promises 99% accuracy at 7-10 weeks (costs $79-$149): https://www.amazon.com/SneakPeek-Early-Gender-Prediction-Test/dp/B016201HCG.

However, both Dory and Sarah noted that with respect to both sex selection and adult onset diseases, IVF and pre-implantation genetic diagnosis (PIGD) are the more common routes to exercise a degree of control. Though not the focus here, consumer offerings such as home gender tests and direct-to-consumer genetic kits along with PIGD all make me wonder about consumer expectations and how they too shape the culture and practices of prenatal care – especially perhaps among affluent and/or well-insured populations. I also wonder about the emphasis U.S. society places on biological parenthood, and about the lengths – financial, emotional, logistical – that some will go to become biological parents.[8] I do not want to minimize the human longing for children, nor the pain that comes from infertility (Harwood 2007). Yet, I wonder if being a biological parent is a human right? Do we need to do more collective and individual reflection on the role of grieving and the reality of limits – physiological, financial, existential? Do we need to keep expanding our understandings of what parenthood means, what "family" means – unhinging it from the necessity of a biological connection?

Insights from three genetic counselors and connections to the larger social context

Demographics

In the U.S., there are approximately 3,500 practicing genetic counselors. Of these, 36 percent work in University Medical Centers, 17 percent work in private hospital/medical facilities and another 17 percent work in public contexts. In terms of specialization, 29 percent work in prenatal care, 25 percent in cancer, and 13 percent in pediatric. Another 33% work in other areas: labs, administration, education, cardiology, neurogenetics, adult genetics, personal genomics, preconception, newborn screening, etc. Over 73 percent of genetic counselors have a Master's degree in Genetic Counseling and/or Genetics (NSGC 2012, 1-13).

The vast majority of genetic counselors identify as non-Hispanic white women. In a 2012 survey conducted by the National Society of Genetic Counselors, of 1339 respondents, 1281 identified as female and 58 as male. In

---

8   Dory commented how she is now seeing women who are 44, 45, 46 years old using IVF and their own eggs – who are pregnant, but have a lot of health issues and prenatal concerns, that would never have been accepted as IVF patients 5 or 10 years ago. Her point was that fertility doctors are now working with older women, and with women who are not as good IVF candidates, and whom they would have turned away a few years ago.

terms of race-ethnicity, 1236 identified as white (92%); while 15 individuals identified as Black, 62 as Asian, 2 as American Indian, 5 as Pacific Islander or Native Hawaiian, and 19 as "other". In terms of age, 1,100 of the 1,338 respondents indicated that they are between 25-44 years old (Ibid., 10f.)

Following Institutional Review Board (IRB) approval, I spoke with seven genetic counselors. Here, I discuss the insights of three individuals – Sarah Morgan, Abby Taylor, and Dory Marlin (all pseudonyms) who work in distinct clinical contexts. None speaks for all genetic counselors or for their profession. Yet, they offer illuminative insight worthy of attention.

Sarah Morgan has worked in genetic counseling since 2009 and has worked in two different clinical contexts. Abby Taylor has been a genetic counselor for 24 years and has worked at the same place for that entire time. Dory Marlin has worked as a genetic counselor for 17 years and she too has stayed at the same site this entire time. Sarah and Dory work almost exclusively in prenatal genetics and see approximately 15-20 prenatal patients a week, whereas Abby sees just 3 prenatal patients per week on average, currently spending about 15 percent of her time in prenatal with the majority of her time spent working in adult genetics clinical services.

All identify as non-Hispanic, white women. Abby speaks Spanish fluently; Sarah speaks a bit of Spanish and Dory understands some Spanish. All make use of translators when needed – preferably in person, but at times they all have to rely on phone translators. Sarah noted that sometimes patients refuse to have a translator present.

All work with diverse populations in terms of race-ethnicity, language of origin, socio-economic class, and insurance coverage. However, Sarah said that in her current employment her patient population is more educated and more likely to be privately insured than in her previous workplace. In her present site, she estimates that 20-30 percent of her patients are insured by Medicaid, whereas at the prior clinic 70-80 percent were Medicaid patients (Phone conversation, 1/6/2014). In contrast, very few of Abby's patients have any private insurance – the vast majority are either uninsured or have Medicaid. Of the three counselors, Abby is the only one to see a significant number of uninsured patients. Dory estimates that 40 percent of her patients are on Medicaid with the other 60 percent being insured by either PPO or HMO insurance.

I first wanted to know how patients find their way into genetic counseling offices. All commented that in the great majority of cases, a physician refers the patient. Sarah explains, "[P]atients mostly find us through their referring obstetrician [...] either to have a conversation about screening and testing options in general or because they've been found to be high-risk for whatever reason – a family history, an ultrasound anomaly, an abnormal screen

(Interview, 9/23/13)." I asked Sarah if patients come knowing what they might or might not want or if they have very little prior knowledge about why they are in her office and what they might want to do or not do. She replied:

> I would say it varies on your institution. So in my current institution, patients generally have a pretty good idea what they're coming in for and what they want, and they may have some questions about other options, but they have a pretty good of idea of "This is why I'm here, this is what I want to do and let's move forward." With my previous place of employment that was definitely *not* the case and it was much more exploratory and patients had far less understanding of why they were coming to see me, which created a lot of [...] unnecessary anxiety for them. (Interview, 9/23/13)

I also wondered how long the professional relationship lasts. All three explained that they normally see patients once or twice in prenatal contexts. A few counseling relationships – when initial screening or testing results reveal a concern – may extend to three or four consults. They each spoke about how they are trained to attend to intense, brief, and stressful moments in patients' lives.

Barriers to Patient Agency

I asked each of the counselors to reflect upon what obstacles get in the way of providing the kind of prenatal care to which they aspire. They raised four issues that frustrate optimal patient care. Perhaps the most obvious barrier is cost. Genetic testing can be expensive ($300-$3,000) depending on the number and kinds of tests performed along with the kind of insurance coverage the patient has – copays, deductibles, if the lab accepts Medicaid insurance or not, etc. All three identified financial costs as a barrier for some. Dory commented that she often spends half of a 1 hour consultation just going over the financial dimensions – what different tests will cost the particular patient depending on her/their specific insurance plan. In contrast, in her current employment, Sarah does not go into detail on the financial aspects of the costs of various tests, other than giving a brief overview and saying that they cannot guarantee insurance coverage.

One of my assumptions going into this work was that Medicaid patients would be at a disadvantage in terms of what they could afford and what Medicaid would cover. Both Abby and Dory stressed that, up to the new cell-free screen, Medicaid has been more than adequate – that they actually prefer Medicaid to some forms of HMO insurance. Second is the matter of timing – if women do not come in for prenatal care in their first trimester – and there are various reasons why women may not (financial, emotional, not knowing they are pregnant, fear, etc.) – they miss out being able to consider having the first trimester screens.

Third, Abby reflected on the institutional challenges regarding where she works and on the social challenges of her patients. In terms of the latter, she remarked that, "Genetics instantly falls low on the list when you know meeting daily needs is a big concern. And that includes transportation to the hospital" (Interview, 12/10/2013). With respect to institutional challenges, she talked about not having private rooms for consultation or enough chairs, along with the sometimes indifferent attitudes of some of the nurses and physicians with whom she works. Recall that most of Abby's patients are either uninsured or insured by Medicaid.

Fourth, and particularly complicated, is the constellation of cultural and educational dynamics. Each of them spends significant time educating others – not only patients, but other health professionals including MDs – about the role and expertise of genetic counselors. They all commented on how little many people know about their profession or what they contribute to patient care. Dory and Abby expressed surprise that this reality has not changed more during the 17 and 24 years of their working life, respectively.

Specifically in terms of counselling patients, all three spoke to the challenges of conveying complex genetic information to patients. Sarah commented that she encounters this with patients of any socio-economic background. Yet, all three noted that at times it can particularly challenging due to linguistic, cultural, and educational barriers. Abby and Dory both explicitly recognize the challenges represented by the homogeneity among their professional ranks. Dory remarked that, "When you talk about culture bumps and [...] evaluating for bias – it's really challenging when you're all the same person" (Interview, 10/15/2013). Abby emphasized that the National Society of Genetic Counselors is aware of this reality and prioritizes the recruitment of graduate students of various races and cultural backgrounds.

Yet, significant educational, racial, and cultural dynamics undeniably can impede understanding and relationship building. As noted earlier, there is a lot of misunderstanding about how screenings are different from diagnostic tests. They also deal with misconceptions regarding what an amniocentesis is (that it injects a needle into the spine of the baby), what causes Down syndrome (smoking pot). Abby lamented, "Oh. There are times when it's just hopeless" (Interview, 10/1/2013).

Abby emphasized that it is not because her patients are unintelligent, but because the information is so technical and also because many of her patients have no interest in hearing it. She elaborated:

My patients are heavily weighted on the Spanish-speaking side. So I see a lot of patients who really had no interest in ever talking to me. And in fact, some of them are a little bothered because some people think that if we start talking about what might happen, it's more likely to happen. (Interview, 10/1/2013)

I asked Abby how she breaks through these cultural barriers. She replied:

I don't, if they, I mean ... I talk to them very briefly and let them know, I try to be reassuring and let them know that most women in their situation have normal healthy babies. Um, that, you know, there's testing that's available but it's completely optional. And if ... they're willing to listen a little bit I try to give them a little bit of a framework, you know, this is, you know, how big the risk is, this is how, you know, and it will continue to increase gradually, but most women in your situation have healthy babies. And if that's all they want to hear ... then that's fine. I don't try to push it beyond that. And sometimes they don't want to hear *that* much. (Interview, 10/1/2013)

All three professionals spoke of the familiar occurrence of having significant number of patients who do not want to be in their office, who do not want the info, who are worried that the appointment will jinx something, and who think that the goal of genetic counselors is to talk them into an abortion if there is a genetic anomaly. Dory explained that in her context she does not see many "worried well" (as I had been during my pregnancy) patients:

There's not a lot of people coming in here like, "I'll pay for anything. I want everything" ... not a lot of high anxiety patients which is so great because most of the patients are very grateful for the information that we have for them ... And ... some of them avoid coming in because they have some ideas about what genetic counseling is. But of course the ones that are the hardest to get in the room are usually the ones that are worried the most. And those are the ones that we can benefit the most. If we get them in the room, by the end of the session they're like, "Oh, ok, this was good, I am glad I did this". (Interview, 10/15/2013)

Dory's hope is that they leave with a better understanding of the possibilities, what the various options offer, and with more overall understanding.

Similarly, I asked Abby what she loves about her job. She responded: "I also just love that it's helping people who desperately need help, who you know are in really dire often, or tough circumstances with what they're coping with and the way they're living." Dory described her role as being a crisis counselor, offering expertise and empathy, and striving to be helpful. At one point, Dory remarked: "It's not we're pro-abortion, but we're 'pro the patient deciding'" (Interview, 12/10/2013).[9]

---

9   Dory commented that the big question that people need to think about in an initial genetic counseling session is not whether or not they would ever consider abortion. Rather, "The

In summary, when I asked them to describe their vocational purpose, the themes of education, empowerment, empathetic decision-making, patient advocacy, and helpful support in a stressful time came up repeatedly. They each said that in general they do not mind if patients make decisions that are different from what the counselor might have elected to do. What matters to them is that they have good information in making whatever decision they make.

They all readily acknowledged that there is significant grey area with regard to many congenital conditions – that they cannot give patients definitive answers in many cases about what the baby's life will be like. Still, they think they can give them helpful things to know and think about so that they can try to discern what realities they can cope with – emotionally, financially, in terms of childcare and educational needs, etc. They also spoke of the importance of giving patients resources for speaking with or reading about others who have made various decisions, through websites, support groups, former patients, or collections of narratives from women who have children with disabilities and others who had abortions.

Dory and Abby also spoke of the value of their profession in its unique expertise – that they, unlike doctors, take time to have these complicated conversations and that they have the training to best explain and interpret what the various tests and results mean. Both discussed how little genetics background most MDs have and that they spend far less time listening to patients and are more directive as a profession – they give opinions, medical advice, order tests, summarize results/next steps.

Returning to my central question, what will bolster moral agency with respect to genetic testing, I would like to offer an insight that came up in conversations with Abby. I asked Abby what – if she had unlimited resources and could dictate policy – would be the ideal role that genetic counseling would play during prenatal care? Her response gave me a new way of thinking about ways forward: "Well, it would begin before conception because really the biggest public health issue I think is folic acid [...] Yeah, and so many of our patients don't know, I mean, most of our patients don't know anything about it. They really have never heard of this." (Interview, 10/1/2013)

Why do I choose folic acid to talk about as a way forward in thinking about moral agency, prenatal care and genetics? Because preconception and prenatal education along with folic acid center the discussion squarely on health and healthcare inequalities with which U.S. society has an obligation to grapple. To reduce one's risk of having a genetic abnormality in pregnancy, ACOG

---

big question you need to get to at some point during the session is 'If the baby has a genetic problem, do you want to know it during the pregnancy?'" (Interview, 10/15/13)

recommends a number of measures, including *not only* prenatal screening, but the use of folic acid, refraining from smoking, drinking or taking illegal drugs, being careful with medications, avoiding infections and exposure to toxins, reducing weight before pregnancy (ACOG 2018). In short, we need to put prenatal genetics into the larger context of U.S. social and health inequity. To illustrate this point, consider a few statistics.

Recall the above statistics on U.S. infant mortality. In 2015, the infant mortality rate for non-Hispanic white infants was 4.82, 5.20 for infants identified as Hispanic, and a shocking 11.73 for Black, non-Hispanic infants – over twice as high as the rate for non-Hispanic whites (Murphy 2017). Every year, over twice as many Black infants die before their first birthday than white infants (Ibid.).

The picture for mothers is also alarming. The U.S. has the highest rate of maternal mortality among industrialized peers, and the number of maternal deaths is rising even as it declines elsewhere. Annually, 700-900 women die from "pregnancy or childbirth-related causes, and some 65,000 nearly die [...]" (Martin/Montagne 2017a). Sixty percent of these deaths are preventable (Ibid.). Again, the racial disparity is startling: Black women are three to four times more likely to die as a result of complications related to pregnancy and/or childbirth than white women.[10] "Put another way, a black woman is 22 percent more likely to die from heart disease than a white woman, 71 percent more likely to perish from cervical cancer, but 243 percent more likely to die from pregnancy- or childbirth-related causes." (Martin/Montagne 2017b) Being pregnant is quite literally life-threatening for Black women.

Racism is a root problem with which the U.S. must contend. ProPublica and NPR collected over 200 stories from Black mothers in 2017. A recurring theme is how unconscious bias affects their care and makes them feel disrespected by medical providers:

> The young Florida mother-to-be whose breathing problems were blamed on obesity when in fact her lungs were filling with fluid and her heart was failing. The Arizona mother whose anesthesiologist assumed she smoked marijuana because of the way she did her hair. The Chicago-area businesswoman with a high-risk pregnancy who was so upset at her doctor's attitude that she changed OB-GYNs in her seventh month, only to suffer a fatal postpartum stroke. Over and over, black women told of medical providers who equated being African American with being poor, uneducated, noncompliant and unworthy. (Ibid.)

---

10   Per the CDC, the pregnancy-related morality rate for Black women was 43.5 vs. 12.7 for white women from 2011-2013 (CDC 2018b).

Regardless of fame (e.g. Serena Williams[11]), education level, socio-economic class, or profession, Black women are too often not believed or heard at key moments in their healthcare.

There also is the matter of insurance or a lack thereof, and prenatal care. Significant numbers of women do not receive sufficient basic prenatal care, let alone adequate information regarding genetic testing options. In highlighting these kinds of realities, I am following the lead of Loretta Ross and other scholars and activists of color who call for moving away from "pro-life vs. pro-choice" dichotomies to prioritize reproductive justice. Loretta Ross and Rickie Solinger explain:

> At the heart of reproductive justice is this claim: all fertile persons and persons who reproduce and become parents require a safe and dignified context for these most fundamental human experiences. Achieving this goal depends on access to specific, community-based resources including high-quality health care, housing and education, a living wage, a healthy environment, and a safety net for times when these resources fail. Safe and dignified fertility management, childbirth, and parenting are impossible without these resources. (Ross/Solinger 2017, 9)

Rather than ask abstractly "Is prenatal genetics ethical or not?", a reproductive justice framework helps us situate the topic within the larger social, racial, and economic context of U.S. medical care for women. And in so doing, it presses us to give focused and sustained attention to longstanding, unjust inequities.

Calling for strong attention to social determinants of health does *not* mean that genetics doesn't matter or that there is no need for prenatal genetic testing/counseling. Rather, the point is that instead of narrowly focusing on prenatal genetics in the abstract ("Is it ethical or not?"), we need to situate it within a larger context of prenatal (and pre-conception) medical care and women's health. Simply put, *both* a woman's genetic makeup *and* her social location (e.g. racial-ethnic, socio-economic class) hold vital information about her specific health risks. Putting these diverse factors into conversation can contribute to a fuller analysis of her health and needs.

Moreover, if more women and girls have access to high quality, comprehensive, attuned and caring healthcare and reproductive education *before* pregnancy, they may be more equipped to negotiate questions and options related to prenatal genetics when/if they later become pregnant. Reproductive

---

11   Serena Williams tells her postpartum story in Vogue (February 2018). Online: https://www.vogue.com/article/serena-williams-vogue-cover-interview-february-2018.

justice demands that *all* women – across race and class lines – are empow-
ered with the agency, support and information needed to be captains of their
own lives – to make reproductive decisions and to parent children in safe and
healthy environments.

Connections to Christian Norms & Worldviews

Genetic testing will continue to be seen and used as key to both pre-conception
and prenatal care for the majority of Americans. Given this fact, the question is
how best to educate ourselves and one another about the options. Dory wants
all of her patients to reflect on "What information do I really want to have
and why?" I would add that asking this question before getting pregnant or
before using assisted reproductive technologies of any kind is important. As
in end of life care, the best time to reflect on what we value in our living and
relations and discuss what we might want or not want is *before* medical providers ask us to think through these hard questions in a time-pressured context. How do faith convictions shape our living and our dying? What does the
vocation of parenthood mean? We cannot know everything until the moment
arises when we have to work through it in real time. Yet, by reading, talking,
reflecting about such questions over time, we can come to know more about
ourselves and our spouse or partner. Perhaps discussion of prenatal genetic
testing should become as much staples in premarital pastoral counseling as
they are in prenatal clinic appointments.

Again, questions and scenarios will remain abstract until they viscerally
are not any more – we become pregnant, we learn that we are a carrier for a
genetic condition – and even in these moments, there is still abstraction. The
abstraction lessens if and when a baby is born, but even then, answers are not
immediately available in all cases about what any child's future or potential
holds. Thus, we have to keep learning to live with the tension of not knowing
and not being in control, even as we can do some things to foster our own and
others' health and well-being. And here is where Christian ethics and theology have much to teach us – about living in the tension of uncertainty and of
accepting undetermined futures, while we also root ourselves in the promise
of divine, ever-present, and unfailing love and grace.

Moreover, I am deeply rooted in Christian liberation perspectives that rail
against what physician and anthropologist Paul Farmer calls "stupid deaths"
(Farmer 2005, 152) and, I would add, "stupid inequalities" in women's health,
public health, and prenatal care. Christian ethical reflection can open our
moral fields of vision to see anew, and of our social and moral obligations to

attend to the common good and prioritize a preferential option for those who do not easily get the prenatal care that others of us take for granted.

How might pre- and postnatal care change if we genuinely value the lives of women and children? First, we who generally experience good birth outcomes and who can access excellent healthcare, especially those who identify as white, need to listen deeply to people who too often do not. Second, in light of what we hear, together as a society, we need to support mothers comprehensively, e.g. funding adequate new parent classes, affordable childcare and other social safety nets.

Indeed, regardless of what one thinks about prenatal genetic testing, there is much we can and ought to do to improve pre-conception and prenatal care: Information about and administration of folic acid, development of better and earlier reproductive education programs for young women – and men. The question for people of faith is this: Will we press further to open our sacred places – houses of worship, college campuses, religious institutions – for robust, honest, open-ended conversations and information?

In addition, we need richer categories that move us beyond the narrow binaries of choice vs. life and an overly heavy reliance on a relatively thin conceptualization of autonomy (a.k.a. informed consent of an individual). Reproductive justice and agency are better formulations because they attend to the myriad social relationships in which any moral decision is rooted. They help us explore what enables women to feel and know they have the capacity to make particular decisions and direct the courses of their own lives and what frustrates such capacity. Again, Christian understandings of the common good may be helpful.

Finally, a common responsibility could unite those concerned with abortion rates in light of genetic testing and those not as troubled by them: Rather than place all the burden on a woman, a couple, or a family to welcome a child with disabilities, we all need to keep looking in the mirror. What, as people of faith, are we doing to ensure that our society makes competent childcare, various therapies, and educational resources readily available to all? Will we pay more taxes to fund them? Will we encourage government policies to do so? Will we support the robust enforcement of the Americans with Disabilities Act? In all, how do we concretely embody authentic welcome of disability, difference, and diversity?

If we defend the right to choose, we have to make sure that all choices are viable. And if we are more pro-life, then we have to ever expand the radar screen of what is considered a prolife issue to include social programs, anti-poverty campaigns, improvement in prenatal care and reproductive education programs. I think faith communities of moral deliberation can help society to reflect on how we all share in a responsibility to raise the next generations of society, to teach future parents how to parent, to work against the structural inequalities that make life – from conception to death – so much harder and so much less fair for large numbers of people. Again, the preferential option for the poor takes center stage. There is much we can do together to improve prenatal care and pre-prenatal care in terms of women's health, infant mortality rates, public health and moral agency so that genetic testing is not seen – or used – as the golden ticket to healthy babies.

Which social structures, professional practices, and theological-ethical frameworks will enable human agency and also help people reckon with inescapable finitude? Theological reflection, as Allen Verhey notes, offers rich tools for wrestling with human responsibility in the context of potent powers and definite limits (Verhey 2003). Faith traditions help us live responsibly and creatively in this existential reality. And they testify to the fact that the more deeply we can live into this paradox, the closer we approach understanding ourselves and others as Imago Dei and the closer we come to knowing our place in this particular moment and world in which we live.

Bibliography

Becker, Amy J. (2011): A good and perfect gift, Ada/MI: Bethany House Publishers.

Brody, Jane E. (2013): Breakthroughs in prenatal screening, in: *The New York Times* 10/07/2013. Online: https://well.blogs.nytimes.com/2013/10/07/breakthroughs-in-prenatal-screening/?_r=0 (last access 04/10/2019).

Browning, Melissa (2014): Risky marriage, Lanham/MD: Lexington Books.

Cahill, Lisa S. (2005): Theological bioethics, Washington/DC: Georgetown University Press.

Centers for Disease Control and Prevention (CDC) (2018a): Data & statistics on birth defects. Online: https://www.cdc.gov/ncbddd/birthdefects/data.html (last access 04/02/2019).

Centers for Disease Control and Prevention (CDC) (2018b): Pregnancy Mortality Surveillance System. Online: https://www.cdc.gov/reproductivehealth/maternalinfanthealth/pmss.html (last access 04/10/2019).

Centers for Disease Control and Prevention (CDC) (2018c): What are birth defects? Online: https://www.cdc.gov/ncbddd/birthdefects/facts.html (last access 04/02/2019).

Centers for Disease Control and Prevention (CDC) (2019): Infant Mortality. Online: https://www.cdc.gov/reproductivehealth/maternalinfanthealth/infantmortality.htm (last access 02/04/2019).

Dollar, Ellen P. (2012): No easy choice, Louisville/KY: Westminster John Knox Press.

Ellison, Katherine/Martin, Nina (2017): Nearly dying in childbirth. Why preventable complications are growing in the U.S., in: NPR 12/22/2017. Online: https://www.npr.org/2017/12/22/572298802/nearly-dying-in-childbirth-why-preventable-complications-are-growing-in-u-s (last access 04/01/2019).

Farmer, Paul (2005): Pathologies of power, Berkeley/CA: University of CA Press.

Greenfieldboyce, Nell (2015): DNA blood test gives women a new option for prenatal screening, in: NPR 01/26/15. Online: https://www.npr.org/sections/health-shots/2015/01/26/368449371/dna-blood-test-gives-women-a-new-option-for-prenatal-screening (last access 04/10/2019).

Harwood, Karey (2007): The infertility treadmill, Chapel Hill/NC: University of NC Press.

Martin, Nina/Montagne, Renee (2017a): The last person you'd expect to die in childbirth, in: ProPublica/NPR 05/12/2017. Online: https://www.propublica.org/article/die-in-childbirth-maternal-death-rate-health-care-system (last access 03/27/2019).

Martin, Nina/Montagne, Renee (2017b): Nothing prevents black women from dying in pregnancy and childbirth, in: ProPublica and NPR 12/07/2017. Online: https://www.propublica.org/article/nothing-protects-black-women-from-dying-in-pregnancy-and-childbirth (last access 03/27/2019).

Mathews, T.J./MacDorman, Marian F./Thoma, Marie E. (2015): Infant mortality statistics from the 2013 period. Linked birth/infant death data set, in: National vital statistics reports 64, 9. Online: https://www.cdc.gov/nchs/data/nvsr/nvsr64/nvsr64_09.pdf (last access 04/02/2019).

Mayo Clinic (2018): Prenatal cell-free DNA screening. Online: https://www.mayoclinic.org/tests-procedures/noninvasive-prenatal-testing/about/pac-20384574 (last access 04(10(2019).

Murphy, Sherry L. (2017): Deaths. Final data for 2015, in: National Vital Statistics Reports 66, 6. Online: https://www.cdc.gov/nchs/data/nvsr/nvsr66/nvsr66_06.pdf (last access 03/27/2019).

Rettner, Rachael (2014): US ranks behind 25 other countries in infant mortality, in: LiveScience, 09/24/2014. https://www.livescience.com/47980-us-infant-mortality-full-term-babies.html (last access 03/27/2019).

Ross, Loretta J./Solinger, Rickie (2017): Reproductive justice, Oakland/CA: University of CA Press.

Scharen, Christian/Vigen, Aana M. (2011): Ethnography as Christian theology and ethics, New York/NY: Continuum, 2011.

The Amercian College of Obstetricians and Gynecologists (ACOG)/Society for Maternal-Fetal Medicine (SMFM) (2016): Ob-Gyns release revised recommandations on screening and testing for genetic disorders. Online: https://www.acog.org/About-ACOG/News-Room/News-Releases/2016/

Ob-Gyns-Release-Revised-Recommendations-on-Screening-and-Testing-for-Genetic-Disorders (last access 04/02/2019).

Verhey, Allen (2003): Reading the bible in the strange world of medicine, Grand Rapids/MI: Eerdmans.

Vigen, Aana M. (2006). Women, inequality, and healthcare. New York/NY: Palgrave.

Responding from the Place of Suffering

Informed Consent and Non-invasive Prenatal Genetic Screening

Michael McCarthy

Introduction

Given the prenatal challenges faced by racial minorities in the United States, prenatal screenings offer an important source of medical information provided that the information from these screens are delivered in an appropriate way. The goal of these screenings is informative and presents patients with medical decisions based on the results. One such screen offered more widely are non-invasive prenatal screenings (NIPS). NIPS screens for Trisomy, 13, 18, and 21.

As Vigen notes in the previous chapter, Latina women face unique challenges in evaluating the results of prenatal screens even with the assistance of genetic counselors. NIPS screens, while morally neutral, require a moral decision from patients should they test positive for one of the above chromosomal anomalies. In order to make this decision, patients need to be offered enough information to make an informed choice. Yet, an informed choice can be difficult given that lack of diversity among prenatal counselors that can speak to patient concerns.

Informed consent after a positive screen for Trisomy 21, Down syndrome, should move from an individualist model of autonomy to a principled autonomy that allows the patient to explore the decision from her reality. This shift would need to incorporate the medical facts, understanding the risks and benefits, and learning from those faced previously with similar decisions. This chapter begins, first, by describing non-invasive prenatal genetic screening. Secondly, it explores what constitutes informed consent through an individual/utilitarian model of autonomy and juxtaposes that with principled autonomy grounded in Ada María Isasi-Díaz's *mujerista* hermeneutic, *lo cotidiano*. The chapter concludes by drawing on both insights from minority participants in clinical research and parents of a child with Trisomy 21 in order to enhance the process for informed consent. Better understanding the reality of the patient and explaining the potential options in a way that prioritizes the patient's reality allows her to make a responsible and informed decision.

© BRILL SCHÖNINGH, 2022 | DOI:10.30965/9783657715428_013

Prenatal Screening Recommendations

Vigen raises concerns regarding the disparities among prenatal health for white women when compared to women of color in the United States. Among the routine recommendations, prenatal care for all women includes prenatal screening and diagnostic tests when necessary. Most prenatal screenings consist of a blood draw in the first and or second trimester. If those screens are positive, further testing, such as amniocentesis or chorionic villus samplings, could be requested. In addition to routine screenings, non-invasive prenatal screening (NIPS) allows for targeted screens that offer a strong positive predictive value for Trisomy 21, Down syndrome (Leonard 2017, 125). Non-invasive prenatal genetic screening (NIPS) has become a routine aspect of prenatal care for high-risk mothers, women over 35 years of age. The American College of Obstetricians and Gynecologists (ACOG) and the National Society of Genetic Councilors (NSGC) recommend that all high-risk pregnant women receive NIPS screening. While other technology is being developed for more targeted genetic testing, the non-invasive prenatal genetic screening focuses specifically on chromosomal aneuploidy.

A chromosomal aneuploidy results in three common types of mutations that NIPS screens for, trisomy 13, 18, and 21. Trisomy 13, or Patau Syndrome, is a mutation that results in several physical and intellectual limitations. The survivability rate beyond the first year that is less than 10%. Trisomy 18 is more common in girls, does not result often in a live birth, and if she lived to term she would likely suffer postpartum complications due to cardiovascular irregularities and multi-organ failure (Witters et al. 2011, 15-17). Given the low survivability of these other diagnoses, this chapter is going to focus on the most survivable mutation, Trisomy 21.

Down syndrome is the most common divergence, affecting 14.2 out of 10,000 live births. NIPS allow for better accuracy in its screening. 99% of pregnancies with a baby that has trisomy 21 can be identified accurately in the first trimester, compared to only 79% in the routine first-trimester screenings (Leonard 2017, 125). Children with Down syndrome can live a relatively healthy life; therefore, the counseling and decision for many pregnant patients is an important one.

82% of parents who receive a diagnosis of Trisomy 21 can remember the exact words of their physician 21 years later. (Skotko et al 2011, 2335). For Latino patients, they tend to rely on the recommendation of the physician, heightening the importance for clear communication that offers the patient the full range of options (Matthew 2012, 164). However, the conversations around the results of testing are generally brief. As Vigen notes, for women of color the conversation takes place in a way that may not speak to a reality or cultural perspective that truly informs the patient of the decision she is making. In a recent study, 63% of women with "abnormal markers" "had no clear understanding of the screening test they had completed and thus had no idea how to interpret abnormal results" (Colicchia et al. 2016, 1151). These results are more disconcerting given that pre and post screening results were discussed with the patient. Given the prevalence of screenings, the lack of clarity around screening results, and the seriousness of the decision being made: How can a patient in this situation make a truly informed decision? From an ethical perspective, the ability to offer informed consent is even further complicated by the rationale for offering non-invasive prenatal screening at no cost to patients.

In 2000, a comparative study between the United States and England discovered that, prior to NIPS, if prenatal genetic screening was offered to over 99% of pregnant women, then at least 56-65% of those with Trisomy 21 needed to be reduced in successive generations to offset the costs of paying for prenatal screening (Leach 2015, 21). Leach's research demonstrates the prevalence of utilitarian thinking behind the use of prenatal genetic screening, "based in part on identifying more pregnancies carrying a child with Down syndrome and then avoiding those costs through abortion" (Leach, 25). NIPS itself is a morally neutral test and can provide valuable information to the mother. However, it takes on a different character if tests are provided with a preference biased for reduction in order for the screening to be financially viable. Given the rationale for free screening, Vigen's argument about the injustices of prenatal care for vulnerable populations raises further concerns about informed consent for a patient with a positive NIPS for Trisomy 21. Whose values and perspectives are prioritized when promoting the importance of prenatal genetic screening amongst vulnerable populations in U.S.? How can better genetic counseling and prenatal care be considered of equitable value and importance in offering resources to support the patient's right to informed consent? A true process of informed consent must offer patients information in a way that responds to their questions of value and meaning.

Informed Consent and *lo cotidiano*

Informed consent is the gold-standard of medical decision making. It entails the patient not only giving permission for, but understanding both the benefits and burdens of treatment options. Informed consent requires a relationship between the health care provider – physician, nurse, genetic counselor, etc. – and the patient built on mutual trust and respecting the autonomy of the patient. Yet, Onora O'Neill notes, "what is grandly called 'patient autonomy' often amounts simply to a right to choose or refuse treatments on offer, and the corresponding obligations of practitioners not to proceed without the patients' consent" (O'Neill 2002, 37). While she does not underestimate the foundational practice of consent, she challenges whether this thin description of autonomy that rests on medical facts alone is sufficient. This thin description of the patient's right to accept or refuse treatment when applied to NIPS proves problematic if only the medical choice is explained.

Informed consent as the right to choose or refuse treatment following a positive screen for Trisomy 21 is more complex. First, if the screening was offered for free, the research demonstrates that is based on a cost benefit analysis that half of women will choose to abort. Second, while abortion is a medical option in certain settings, the burden of ensuring that the decision process is truly informed requires a description of the choice that extends beyond the medical facts. Informed consent requires an attempt to understand the meaning and values from which the patient is making the decision. Given Vigen's reservations and narrative accounts, which further research supports, the post screening conversations tend to be brief and unremarkable (Colicchia et al. 2016, 1151). Thus, how can a more robust process of informed consent be developed for patient's from medically vulnerable population after a positive screen for Trisomy 21? What description of the risks and benefits going forward would allow for a reasonable understanding of what it might be like to parent a child with Down syndrome? Are support systems, regardless of choice, made known to the patient to assist in her decision-making process? Given the power dynamics between the patient and the provider, the emphasis needs to shift from the medical framework for decision making to consider more seriously the reality of the patient.

While one thinks often of social injustices more broadly, the inequality of patient and provider also creates an imbalance that needs to be addressed justly. Rather than reinforce the power dynamic, beginning and sticking only to the medical facts of the decision, a process of truly informed consent should start from the place and experience of the patient. The place and experience of injustice provides the foundational loci from which one ought to begin ethical conversations (Ellacuría 1990, 386; Isasi-Díaz 2002, 13). Place, moreover, functions as an intellectual category; it reveals one's social position, motivation, the position from which one acts, and for whom one acts. The place from which the free screening is offered is biased already toward terminating the pregnancy, but that is an unknown starting point for the patients making the informed decision. Disclosing the rationale for covering NIPS may not be necessary, if the place of the patient is prioritized first. If the women who are most likely to receive lower quality of care and less explanation are women of color, then greater efforts to ask about her reality are needed. Vigen's chapter not only identifies the weaknesses of the U.S. health care system's attention to the prenatal needs for women of color but also the neglect of understanding – or asking about – their story.

If the heart of informed consent is the freedom to make a decision that understands the risks and benefits of the decision, then that decision needs to be put in a language that offers a more holistic picture beginning with the patient's reality. Ada María Isasi-Díaz describes *mujerista* theology as a birth-centered theology, one that is rooted in the lives of "mothers, sisters, daughters, women lovers, friends" (Isasi-Díaz 2004, 92). Isasi-Díaz's description moves beyond the medical foundation of decision-making to the social network within which decisions are made, the place of *lo cotidiano*. *Lo cotidiano* "constitutes the immediate space of our lives [...] where we meet and relate to that material word that is made up not only of physical realities but also is made up of how we relate to that reality [...] [and] situates us in our experiences" (Ibid., 95). Rather than an exercise in cultural awareness, the hermeneutic of *lo cotidiano* provides a framework for informed consent. By asking about the experience and reality of the patient faced with a difficult decision, it gives life to what can be a sterile and binary choice. Beginning a conversation from *lo cotidiano* creates space for the patient to describe her reality and what is important to her within the context of her community. Conversations that start from *lo cotidiano* recognize that "the poor and oppressed understand and face reality in a different way from that of the powerful and the privileged" (Ibid., 100). It shifts the power dynamic away from the clinical framework and into the place of the patient.

While informed consent often focuses exclusively on the medical facts, Latina patients want a broader context from which their medical decisions are made. In a medical context, however, there is always a concern of introducing bias into the patient's process of decision-making and default to focusing on the medical decisions. Nevertheless, when a counselor or physician is unable to speak to the cultural context of a patient that too introduces a bias into the conversation. While Isasi-Díaz offers a theological perspective, she also offers a practical one that expands the process of informed consent beyond a focus on the medical facts and incorporates the lived experience of the patient.

Towards a Principled Autonomy

O'Neill is helpful in distinguishing between an individual autonomy that aims to maximize happiness and one that integrates other value-based perspectives:

> If we assume a full Utilitarian account of maximizing happiness, we subordinate and marginalize individual autonomy itself; if we do not, the line between harmful and non-harmful action and policies will often be blurred. (O'Neill 2002, 73)

In prenatal genetic screening the focus falls on the autonomous mother to interpret the most likely medical scenarios. Many patients, and in particular minority patients, do not feel that the statistical information alone is sufficient to make an informed decision. O'Neill draws on Kant to describe a principled autonomy that focuses on obligation to individuals and communities as a way to recast the Utilitarian reasoning that frames decisions based on NIPS results.

Rather than focus on a process of informed consent that prioritizes medical information and individual decision making, principled autonomy focuses on values and relationships that shape the individual's right to informed consent. Principled autonomy has a commitment to reject deception, and is expressed through "truthful communication, through care not to mislead, through avoidance of exaggeration, through simplicity and explicitness, through honesty in dealing with others, in a word through trustworthiness" (Ibid., 98). What is missing as a component of NIPS counseling for Latina women is a broader description of what constitutes parenting or carrying a child to term with Trisomy 21. If the child will live with a disability, what support options are available? While the utilitarian offers a clear rationale for offering NIPS, the process for post-screening counseling often lacks the detail and nuance that patient's want and deserve. Principled autonomy, grounded in *lo cotidiano* expands the possibility of more comprehensive and practical approach to informed consent.

Practical Approaches to Informed Consent

Sighted frequently in the limitations around informed consent are language and cultural barriers that restrict a patient's understanding and deference to the health care professionals. Scarce research exists into the process of informed consent in the clinical context for minority patients. However, including minority populations in clinical research does offer avenues for considering better processes for informed consent. (Matthew 2008, 150). Though the goals of clinical research differ from clinical care – producing generalizable knowledge compared to offering treatment that benefits the patients – the desired process for informed consent in clinical research proves translatable to the clinical setting.

A group responsible for recruiting minority participants in research cite three preferred ways to make a decision that offer insights for medical informed consent. First, minority research participants preferred more than one, one on one discussion with the researcher (Quinn et al. 2013, 50). The study participants cited the importance of an initial conversation, but saw the value in follow-up conversations to answer any further questions. Second, they wanted to have take-home information that was easy to understand and language appropriate, some even cited videos as helpful. One of the challenges to meeting this demand is that despite ACOG requiring discussion of adoption with a positive screen for Trisomy 21, it is rarely done. Moreover, 45% describe training on prenatal genetic counseling as barely adequate or non-existent (Leach 2015, 23). Thus, dramatic improvements would need to be made for educational requirements to meet the patient request. Third, potential research participants expressed a desire to talk to other study participants. Thus, analogously to the situation of prenatal genetic counseling, it is not sufficient only to speak to the medical personnel, but to speak to other women that have been faced with a similar prenatal diagnosis. In a certain sense, this expansion would mean offering resources to help a patient understand their new reality post-diagnosis. The expansion of resources and more frequent conversations with the health care provider would better inform the choice the patient is making. In addition, the fact that research participants requested broader conversation with others who had participated suggests that more information from parents of a child with Down syndrome might prove helpful.

In a survey of parents who have a son or daughter with Down syndrome, only 5% express embarrassment by their child and 4% describe regret in having their child. Conversely, 99% report that they love their child, 97% are proud of them, and 79% describe their outlook on life as more positive because of their child (Skotko et al. 2011, 2335). The narrative of these parents places a different value than the one that argues for covering the cost of NIPS based on a need to reduce the number of individuals born with Trisomy 21 by 56-63% within a generation. Beyond the quantitative data, Skotko's study provided the opportunity for qualitative information for parents of future Down syndrome children.

Many parents offered excitement for the life of the future child and the parents. They suggested that that they would be astounded by what their child would accomplish. Others offered advice to the parent/s: "Relax. Take it one day at a time. Your life will be so much richer for having this child in your life."

Another parent notes: "What at first appears to be the worst possible thing that could be happening, can turn into the best possible thing." (Ibid., 2341) The experience of these parents is a much-needed balance to the clinical framing of a positive screen. These narratives capture the choice that a patient faces following a diagnosis of Trisomy 21, and when paired with an offer for further conversations with medical professionals and enhanced resources to take-home, patients have a greater opportunity to make an informed decision that respects the framework of principled autonomy grounded in *lo cotidano*.

Conclusion

The goal of informed consent is rooted in patient understanding the risk and benefits of pursuing one particular course of treatment over another. With the increasing number of prenatal tests and screenings that will continue to be made available, developing a process for informed consent that prioritizes intentionally the wishes and values of patients is essential. Given the disparities that already exist in prenatal care in the U.S., the challenge to offer truly informed consent is even more difficult when the mother receives an unexpected diagnosis about her child.

NIPS provide a helpful resource to detect and decide what course of action the patient wants to pursue. However, the lack of sufficient patient counseling around NIPS makes the likelihood of a process for informed consent grounded in principles of autonomy seem limited. For vulnerable populations, beginning from the experience of the patient is crucial. Isasi-Díaz offers *lo cotidiano* as the place for Latina patients to begin exploring the decision upon receiving a positive screen for Trisomy 21. Given the research on counseling following non-invasive prenatal screening, the health disparities present in the Latina community, informed consent requires that the patient is given the option to explore the decision from her reality (*lo cotidiano*) by incorporating the medical facts, understanding the risks and benefits, and learning from those faced previously with similar decisions.

Bibliography

Colicchia, Laura/Holland, Cynthia/Tarr, Jill/Rubio, Doris/Rothenberger, Scott/ Chang, Judy (2016): Patient-health care provider conversations about prenatal genetic screening: Recommendation or personal choice, in: Obstetrics and Gynecology 127, 6: 1145-1152. Online: https://insights.ovid.com/crossref?an= 00006250-201606000-00023 (last access 03/27/2019).

Ellacuria, Ignacio (1990): Filosofía de la realidad histórica, San Salvador/El Salvador: UCA Editores.

Griffiths, Anthony J.F./Miller, Jeffrey H./Suzuki, David T./Lewontin, Richard C./Gelbart, William M. (2000): An introduction to genetic analysis. 7th edition. New York/NY: W. H. Freeman Aneuploidy. Online: https://www.ncbi.nlm.nih.gov/books/NBK21870/ (last access: 1.05.2018).

Isasi-Díaz, Ada M. (2002): Lo Cotidiano: A key element of mujerista theology, in: Journal of Hispanic/Latino Theology 10, 1: 5-17. Online: https://repository.usfca.edu/cgi/viewcontent.cgi?article=1026&context=jhlt (last access 03/27/2019).

Isasi-Díaz, Ada M. (2004): La Lucha continues: Mujerista theology, Maryknoll/NY: Orbis Books.

Jaramillo, Sonia/Moreno, Socorro/Rodríguez, Viviana (2016): Emotional burden in parents of children with Trisomy 21. Descriptive Study in a Colombian Population. Propiedades psicométricas de la Escala de Ideología de Género en adolescentes colombianos, in: Universitas Psychologica 14, 1: 29-38. Online: http://www.scielo.org.co/pdf/rups/v15n1/v15n1a03.pdf (last access 03/27/2019).

Leach, Mark W. (2015): Unjustified. The imbalance of information and funding with noninvasive prenatal screening, in: AJOB Empirical Bioethics 6, 1: 21-30. Online: https://doi.org/10.1080/23294515.2014.993100 (last access 03/27/2019).

Leonard, Samantha (2017): Current concepts in noninvasive prenatal screening (NIPS), in: Journal of fetal medicine 4, 3: 125-130. Online: https://doi.org/10.1007/s40556-017-0122-6 (last access 03/27/2019).

Matthew, Dayna B. (2008): Race, religion, and informed consent – lessons from social science, in: The journal of law, medicine & ethics 36, 1: 150-173. Online: https://doi.org/10.1111/j.1748-720X.2008.00244.x (last access 03/27/2019).

Quinn, Sandra/Garza, Maria/Butler, James/Fryer, Craig/Casper, Erica/Thomas, Stephen/Barnard, David/Kim, Kevin (2012): Improving informed consent with minority participants. Results from researcher and community surveys, in: Journal of empirical research on human research ethics 7, 5: 44-55. Online: https://doi.org/10.1525/jer.2012.7.5.44 (last access 03/27/2019).

Skotko, Brian G./Levine, Susan P./Goldstein, Richard (2011) Having a son or daughter with Down Syndrome. Perspectives from mothers and fathers, in American journal of medical genetics. Part A 155, 10: 2335-2347. Online: https://doi.org/10.1002/ajmg.a.34293 (last access 03/27/2019).

Witters, G./Van Robays, J./Willekes, C. et al. (2011): Trisomy 13, 18, 21, Triploidy and Turner syndrome: the 5T's. Look at the hands, in: Facts, views & vision in ObGyn 3, 1: 15-21. Online: https://www.ncbi.nlm.nih.gov/pmc/articles/PMC3991414/ (last access 03/27/2019).

PART IV

Spirituality and Religion in Care and Ethical Counselling

Suffering in the Practice of the Christian Faith in God

Ottmar Fuchs

Introduction

When death bursts violently into an active life, when a deadly disease destroys the existing form of self-empowerment in life, then this extreme situation reveals whether faith in God can also keep pace with these experiences. In a very specific, unsurpassable and explosive way, the relationship between power and religion is broken when it encounters the question of what this "power" remaining in the scope of religion actually is, if humans are completely powerless. At the same time, the question arises about what kind of power this is, which, in view of religion, still has a relationship with it, in view of the powerlessness created by violence, disease, and death and beyond, which can be viably supporting, and allows for hope.

Here, the Christian message is, in a specific manner, able to provide information: the Christ's suffering and death are an expression of the love of a God who is capable of empathy. Suffering is not removed from a suffering-free God. The Christian drama of the relationship between love and death, which pervades world literature as a motif and signals in this literary "tip of the iceberg" the central question of human life, is an occurrence of its own, and one which is at the same time highly productive for the life of the believer.

Because God lets suffering get close to Him in Jesus, because "since then" the resurrected Christ keeps the wounds of humankind in God, because the Spirit of Christ continues to "groan" with those who suffer (cf. Rm 8, 26) and mourns because It exists in a lasting historical presence in every suffering person (cf. Mt 25, 42-43), because He does not let the sin of people become boundaries between humankind and God, but goes beyond these boundaries (cf. 1 Jn 4, 10), because He shows substantial and existential solidarity with those who suffer, Christ provides suffering with a "transcendence" into God and, therefore, never separates the transcendence of God from an immanence in the suffering person.

The Christian dealing with suffering, in particular in the fields of disease and dying, of physical and spiritual pain, can be quite contradictory, depending on the situation and person: I will focus, also with biblical excerpts and

© BRILL SCHÖNINGH, 2022 | DOI:10.30965/9783657715428_014

narratives, directly on the God-related speech of faith, on the petition, lament and praise, with varying tension between resistance and surrender.

a)   The *prayer of petition* offers one's own concerns and needs to God and seeks ways of getting out of hardship and/or to overcome it. There is lamenting and weeping as well, not as an accusation, but as an expression of pain and powerlessness, in the hope of being heard. The success of the prayer is, however, unfair to those whose petition does not lead to success. The petition can, in recognition of the sovereignty of God, lead to the surrender to God's will and to his unfathomable mystery.

b)   The *lamentation* to and against God, by contrast, confronts suffering with the love of God, and expresses the difference between promised salvation and experienced affliction. The answers of theology to the theodicy for the justification of God cannot reassure us. 40% of the psalms are texts of conflict and accusation. After such prayers had been criminalized by the church as "quarrelling" for centuries, they are, with the emancipation of believers from ecclesiastical obedience structures, gaining a constantly growing significance, supported by a suffering-sensitive theology, which in turn carries this fundamental conflict into the relationship with God himself (Fuchs 2016).

c)   At the end of the lamentation, there is a praising of God, a *surrendering*, but one which has gone through resistance and has reached a special "maturity". It is this recognition of the mysterious God that is released from any instrumentalization. He is praised for who he is, as the one who brings everything to a good end in an intangible future. This praise of God often occurs counterfactual to current experiences, i.e. it must not be confused with gratitude, but expresses thanks as a promise for a future which does not yet exist.

Invocation: Dialectics of One's Own Wish and God's Will

Trust in the Prayer of Petition

One of the ways of dealing with suffering in religion, and also in Christianity, is the prayer of petition. In the prayer of petition, one asks God for something which is close to one's heart. This uttering of one's own wishes and needs in front of God is a very significant "addressing" of God. On an interpersonal level, it is the worst break in communication to say "I will never ask him/her again for anything!" This also applies to the relationship with God, if one relies on the assumption that what is important to men is also important to Him. In particular, when people wish for something intensively, a sincerity shows itself which should not be excluded from the relationship with God if one wants to come into contact with God with heart and soul, with feelings and wishes, and wants to be taken seriously by Him. Consequently, the prayer of petition also plays a central role in the praying of Jesus (cf. Mt 7, 7-8).

When standing in front of God in a prayer of petition and formulating one's *own will*, there is a vehement description of one's own affliction. This is an act of "will-fulness". At the same time, the verbalization can, however, permit at the same time some distancing from oneself. The rush of aspirations toward God must not yet render the "Thy will be done!" impossible. First of all, it needs to be noted that God also takes people seriously in their obtrusiveness and willfulness (cf. Lk 11, 5f.). One's own "position" must not be withheld or given up. The surrender is not a blind self-submission. It goes through the tension between one's wishes and "Thy will be done".

In relying on being heard, the *freedom of God* is already designed in a way that people are addressed differently, maybe "completely differently", without giving up the hope that, "at the end of the day", He wants what is best, even if one's own wish is not fulfilled, even if this occurs in a completely different manner than one has fantasized about it. To let God be bigger, and also more unfathomable, than one's own petition: this, too, is part of the Christian prayer of petition.

The therapeutic effects of this way of praying should not be underestimated. Whoever elevates wishes and concerns to a dialogue of verbal expression, creates a linguistically and psychologically effective delimitation, a setting, or a framing of what is of concern. Formulated through linguistic awareness, it cannot, like the unspeakable, grow at the base of emotions into mostly unjustified big concerns, making days and nights exceedingly depressing. This applies to big and small everyday concerns as well as to to concerns of conscience, which people have because of their guilt. Such praying reveals that one can again see life and people outside of one's own concerns, so that one bad experience does not overshadow one's whole life and paralyzes constructive acts.

The prayer of petition does not, however, become magic, but is actually a strong relationship, since the relationship is endured and carried forward even if the prayers are not fulfilled. Popular piety has not resulted in a breakdown of the relationship with God, despite all the disappointments and suffering. This relationship is too strong, stronger even than all "if ... then ..."-temptations. This does not preclude that people may lose their faith over the worst experiences of loss, because God has not helped. They then look for other ways outside religion. Or they persevere in the accusation of God, whom they cannot forgive.

Unfavorable Response

It is a question of spirituality, whether something is experienced as an intervention by God, an intervention by response (when a surgical operation is successful and one recovers), or not. Without a doubt, there are evidential experiences which occur between a prayer of petition and an answered prayer, and which belong as such to the core of biblical spirituality. In faith, the response to a prayer is possible; and one cannot deny God intervening either, because this would likewise be an intolerable limit to His freedom. The experience of intervention would, however, become "magical", if one made it a condition for one's relationship with God. Because there are also opposite biblical prayer experiences, namely that God does not answer and remains hidden (cf. Ps 88). One cannot "count" on the intervention of God, here, there is no "if ... then ..."-relationship.

One has to, however, experience that God's intervention appears to be coincidental; one has to expect that one cannot count on Him, that one remains, at the end of the day, dependent on oneself, and that a possible "intervention" by God in turn is experienced as both motivated and unmotivated. If one still adds the thought that God refuses any intervention in certain texts of the bible, and that His "being the Lord" in this life is does not necessarily mean a forceful self-assertion, one may claim as a biblical spirituality a relationship with God in which no intervention is expected anymore, in particular since any salvation or non-salvation reinforces the strong internal dynamics of unfairness.

This is not directed against the experiences of response, which are possible time and again, but is a plea in favor of a spirituality which gratefully accepts the response, and, at the same time, not only accepts it in respect to others, but co-represents their wishes in its prayer, for a spirituality, which can leave the requested intervention of God to God. This spirituality opens itself up to solidarity with all those people who do not experience any salvation. Jesus aligns himself with them, too. He rejects the intervention of God by dying on the cross.

This does not mean that the spirit of God (and hence the power of God) did not have any effect in history, and that there are no criteria for the identification of this power; it does not mean that in this age, however, but not in a self-aggrandizing and arrogant attitude, the act of praying, lamentation and accusation, hope and supplication, gratitude and praise of God are present. At any rate, it would be good for Christianity, after centuries of an often unbridled and often disastrous identification of the "others" of historical and biographical events with the intervention of God (which always excludes those for whom He does not intervene) to have, in this respect, a long moratorium of renunciation. In faith, too, it is possible to consider salvation or non-salvation as a coincidence; nothing has to be identified as intervention of God or His non-intervention. Gratitude and lamentation are possible in both cases because, at the end of the day, God remains responsible for everything that happens in creation, be it in the linguistic game of intervention or in the linguistic game of coincidence (Meier 2012).

Resistance

Lamentation: Resistance and Hope

Lamentation has already been addressed. In the German terminology, it already becomes clear: if I ask somebody for *something*, the claim is directed at the person who is considered as *responsible* for one's condition. In this case there is a request for something, too, i.e. salvation, but in the highly conflicted relationship of a lamentation. This dimension of a relationship crisis and a crisis is not (yet) part of the prayer of petition, or is no longer part of it. To formulate it more strikingly: The supplicant wants *something* from God; the lamentation wants to hold God Himself responsible. The lamentation is a prayed argument with God (Fuchs 1987; Fuchs 1982; Fuchs 2001; Hieke 1998; Janowski 2003). It deals with the apparent disruption of confidence in God as an issue of trust.

The most well-known prayer of lamentation in Christian faith is Psalm 22, with its vehement initial question "My God, my God, why have you abandoned me?" In addressing the question, the crisis is attributed to God, claiming from God what had been promised in terms of salvation and has so far been fulfilled, but is now incomprehensibly and shockingly no longer the case. God has withdrawn.

Jesus prays this psalm in human- and godforsaken distress on the cross (cf. Mk 15, 34). In his deep distress, He relies on a prayer of His people which He has known for a long time, and which is now, at this moment, available to Him as a prayer. It is a demanding prayer resulting from dispair and the feeling of being left alone by God. But nonetheless, it is already an intensive beginning to a relationship with God.

Psalm 22 (abridged, New American Bible, revised edition, excluding the corrections in v. 22b and 23a.)

> 2. My God, my God, why have you abandoned me?
>   Why so far from my call for help,
>   from my cries of anguish? [...]

5. In you our fathers trusted;
    they trusted and you rescued them. [...]
7. But I am a worm, not a man,
    scorned by men, despised by the people. [...]
12. Do not stay far from me,
    for trouble is near,
    and there is no one to help. [...]
15. Like water my life drains away;
    all my bones are disjointed.
    My heart has become like wax,
    it melts away within me.
16. As dry as a potsherd is my throat;
    my tongue cleaves to my palate;
    you lay me in the dust of death. [...]
20. But you, LORD, do not stay far off;
    my strength, come quickly to help me. [...]
22. Save me from the lion's mouth,
    from the horns of the wild bulls – you have heard me.
23. I will proclaim your name to my brethren;
    in the assembly I will praise you.

In a fervent way, the praying person lays out his distress before God. And in the middle of this distress, where a person does not seem to see any way out, the encounter with God releases an enormous power of hope. It is almost incredible that, at this point of disaster, people actually hope against all hope! Praying shows that it is exactly at this point that God "emerges" in the life of a person. In going through the lamentation, in not having to hide one's own situation from God, literally in the deepest valley, the miracle occurs. The lamentation turns into an immediate certainty of response: "You answer me / you are with me / you deliver me!" (Psalm 22, 22b: 'ănîṯānî).

Nothing has happened yet externally, but internally the relationship with God has radically changed. It is not only the belief that God is near when all is well, but also that He is near or even nearer in affliction and suffering. This destroys every talisman-like "Dear Lord", every "if ... then ..." – conflict within the relationship with God, i.e. according to the motto "When I am well, You are near!" or, "If I am close to You in my faith, I should be fine!" God is no longer associated only with wellbeing. Why should one believe now, when one has nothing, no benefit from it?

In the conflicting language of the lamentation, the believer learns to let God be God, and is at the same time given the hope that this sovereign God is always close to him, in particular in the deepest distress. Contrary to facts, people stick to the concept of a "good" God. With the complaint, not only are traditional perspectives of the submission of God to one's own wishes destroyed, but also of the submission to God. In this way, the self-confident a person gains back confidence in God in a different form.

Erich Fromm refers to these psalms as dynamic, because their objective is for the praying person to change. They are texts that leave you altered. "It is the seeming paradox that despair can only be overcome if you have experienced it in its full depth." (Fromm 1980, 168)

For Jesus, too, nothing changes on the cross. God does not intervene, not in His case nor, as it often happens, for humankind. And we do not know why! There is no miracle which takes the distress away. And nonetheless, there is a miracle, namely that the distress prayer to God raises a new and now unconditional trust in God being near in distress, and that the calculation is wrong: wellbeing as a sign of the proximity of God, and distress as a sign of God being distant, although this calculation might always become a temptation.

No Victor's Discourse

God reveals no answers in the sense of an explanatory knowledge, but His co-being with humankind. Faith does not need any victor's discourse. It is not about apology in the sense of wishing to be right in a dogmatist society (Fuchs 2017). Nor does God have to be justified, as Job's friends believe (Jb 3-5).

It is characteristic that, in Psalm 22, the initial question "why" is not answered anywhere. Nor does Jesus provide any explanations of why there is sin and suffering. He rather accompanies those who suffer and stands side-by-side with the sinners. And finally, He claims on the cross, at a place of extreme remoteness from God, the proximity of God. And nonetheless He is rescued. This is embodied by the Christian faith in His resurrection, in His rescue beyond death. For this reason, this psalm has become the prayer mourning of men and women left behind, who followed Jesus between his death and his resurrection. In this way, this prayer of mourning with its hope for rescue becomes a spiritual possibility for our eyes to be actually opened to perceive the epiphany of the crucified Christ and believe in His resurrection (cf. Lk 24, 13-35).

In the confrontation with the immutable, it is easy to identify phases of mourning throughout the lamentation process, and in respect of which, God is petitioned in the prayer as "a companion in mourning and dying". There is shock, then th protest, then the danger of despair and then the breakthrough of a new calm and strength in dedication (Spiegel 1973). This is, however, only possible because rebellion was accepted, because devotion does not prevent resistance, but only materializes in it or after it. Against the backdrop of the unaffirmable disaster that people experience in themselves and/or in others, there is a fight for affirmation which does not know anything and hopes for everything (Werbick 1986, 69 ff.).

In the presence of distress, the believer realizes that God listens and responds. This "response" means: The salvation is already firmly decided in God. It is a reality in God. It is "only" a question of time until the praying person will experience it. The lamentation process as reproduced paradigmatically in Psalm 22, constitutes the concentration of a process which can take minutes, but also days, weeks and years, even decades or a whole life. In the end, it comes true in salvation through the resurrection. The praying person interrupting himself in the middle of the part of the verse of Psalm 22, 22: "From the horns of the wild bulls (i.e. in particular in suffering) – (and then unexpectedly) you answer me, you deliver me (also against all appearances)!" is best characterized by a dash. The time between these two fragments can be a long time of silence, also of loss of faith during which one halts in speaking and does not know how to go on, until speech comes back because one knows how it will go "on". Here, speechlessness and shortage of speech interrupt speech. This is a critical time during which we no longer know how we can still pray.

According to Paul, the Spirit of the Risen Lord vicariously takes over further praying by bridging the silence and reappearance with a sigh, which we cannot express in words because it is itself part of the distress which makes us speechless (cf. Rm 8, 26-27). He prays our prayer, where we can no longer pray, and He even does it on the same level of suffering as the suffering person (i.e. not from a casual remote existence). He can do it because He is the risen *crucified* Christ. He experiences for himself the horror that makes people speechless: but in it He still can find the words to address the Father in our place. For He is the crucified *Risen One*. In this way, the Spirit of God does not only exist in the praying person as long as he speaks, but He stands in for him when he has become speechless: in the face of hardship and the remoteness of God experienced therein. In the latter, the Spirit of the Risen Lord is, with His sigh, likewise still solidary and attributes it to God, as at the time Jesus experiences the forsakenness by God, and prays the beginning of Psalm 22. The incarnate God represents in God the complaint against God. From this perspective, too, the prayer of lamentation is the interactive execution of negative theology (Caspar 1998, 93 f.; Caspar 1998, 124). With Christ, the believers have a power in God to whom they can say everything and lament about everything, without having to fear being sent away as insubordinate or be punished as quarrelling.

Eschatological Event

Most lamentations are not heard on this side. Consequently, the lamentation bridges – in what it demands and in what it hopes for –the boundaries of death. If there is a hope for the victims of history, then it must be assumed that their lamentation does not fall silent upon their death, but that it continues beyond death, as a request to God but above all as an accusation of the perpetrators.

This is the only way to hope for the victims, not only for survival, but for justice, when they can lament before God. In this respect, the resurrection of the dead proves to be a condition for the last (death) cry of the old world, existing at the same time as the first (birth) cry into the new world. The coming judge himself will stand on the side of their lamentation and accusation; He will facilitate and support them in the tribunal of the Last Judgement. The lamentation is, therefore, also an eschatological event, because it hopes that God not only answers with salvation, but will also answer at last the numerous questions of the suffering of humankind. This answer will not be cheap; it must not be below the level of what has been suffered (Fuchs 2018, 67-82).

This answer is that God reveals to us experientially what He has already shown in his incarnate and suffering Son, that He was never remote from us, that He has experienced in Christ the suffering and the lamentations of humankind. We also believe in his omnipotence, which is necessary to share with those who have been suffering throughout history. Whoever has already done this in his life, namely to be with seriously ill people and not run away, knows that this is not a trifle, but that it requires a lot of strength. It is, therefore, possible to imagine that only an all-powerful God can be so close to all people in their suffering, and that He can share it.

In the experience of the worst negativity, the cry for and the accusation against God is not given up. This is not enough, though. This tension is pushed to the limits by means of a very specific prayer, and, at the same time, stretched and relaxed to the infinite: it is the prayer of the praise of God, the doxology. How is it to be understood, provided that one can actually understand it at all?

Dedication to God's Secret

The Doxology as Praise of God
At first sight, lamentation and praise seem to be related to one another in the same way as fire and water. But if one takes a closer look, the prayer of praise does not relate to lamentation in the same way as the prayer of thanksgiving: because the prayer of thanksgiving would not be said in distress. The prayer of praise, however, would. In this third part of Psalm 22, God is praised, and the whole world is called upon to praise God. However, the deplorable situation of the praying person has not changed.[1] It is not in the situation, but in the relationship with God, where everything changes.

---

1   Concerning the change from lamentation to praise in Psalm 22, Verse 22b, although distress has not yet changed (cf. Müller 1996; Schoors 1984).

In going through the lamentation, the relationship with God has, however, changed from accusation to praise. How is this possible?! It is probably the most crazy thing we encounter in biblical prayer. The existing ascriptions are turned upside down: Usually attributing the prayer of praise to a well-being situation, here, this order of spiritual text is thoroughly destroyed. The doxology is not only attributed to the prayer of thanksgiving, but it has now also a related with lamentation!

In Job 1, 21 the mentioned connection is described with hymnal precision: "Naked I came from my mother's womb, And naked I shall return there. The LORD gave and the LORD has taken away. Blessed be the name of the LORD." Out of affliction he succeeds (or rather he is given the blessing) to turn away from himself to the great Creator God, the omnipotent God, who stands above everything, and who is greater than everything (also than the affliction of Job).

Job's word is no indistinct qualification and trivialization of life (meaning that it actually doesn't matter what is given and what is taken away). Here, too, it is not about highlighting God as an arbitrary God who doesn't care how He deals with people. God is not to be made smaller and uglier but greater – greater than one's own misery, so that a possible salvation can exist in God. Doxology allows for faith in God against all evidence.

The human powerlessness experienced by Job is not the last that remains; it remains and is always second-to-last, compared to the actual last, compared to God. Job does not take himself nor his own misery more important than God. Even if it sounds paradoxical: the humility of worship uplifts by still thinking that God is not taken in by the afflictions of humankind, but is with His infinite mystery infinitely more than a person can perceive and experience. Although God is not acting in a wholesome manner, nonetheless, His assumed power to act is praised in creation and history.[2]

Job does not turn his experience of misery into a totalitarian yardstick for the judgement of God. He lets God be greater than everything he experiences. It is a God-empowering praise of God, and redeems humans from self-deification, be it in their powerfulness or powerlessness, by "deifying" their powerlessness in such a way that it and thus death were not equal to the omnipotence of God.

God Is Greater than "Everything"

In doxology, faith is based on the fact that God is neither surpassed what is prayed or thanked for, nor by the suffering. Since, if He were not, in addition to

---

2   Concerning the polarity of might and mercy as the core to the spirituality of praise of the psalms (cf. Steiof 2005).

everything else, all-powerful in an intangible and infinitely mysterious way, we would not have any hope beyond our limited joy, affliction or death.

However, where people accept this presentiment, where they accept it as a blessing, everything is always possible on a large and small scale, as Elie Wiesel narrates in his "Trial of God" (Wiesel 1987). In Shamgorod, the Jewish community meets for the service. Based on their history of persecution, they put God on trial and accuse him (even to a point of condemnation) because he has forsaken his People. As soon as the judgement has been pronounced, the rabbi stands up and invites the community to the most important praise of Israel, the main prayer during the Shabbat celebration, comparable to Job's hymnal praise of God.

The most fascinating thing about this praise is that people, regardless of the situation in which they find themselves, put themselves and their situation aside, and focus on the recognition of the unintelligible, intangible and omnipotent God. In this mystery, which is not easy to relate to current life, which goes beyond all access to God, there is actually hope, in this life and beyond, which is rooted in His mystery, not in our knowledge and actions (Rahner 1980). It is the spirituality of letting go.

In doxology, no "if ... then ..."-game is possible anymore with God, and it is also absolutely unnecessary. If the biblical spirituality is not pointless, but if it actually reveals the direction of the content of this mystery (namely that God in the deepest abyss of His mystery is at the same time the deepest love and salvation) there is no need for any further access. Access exists only in a context with limited resources. In the case of God there are, however, no conditions. This dissolution of boundaries is exactly what doxology draws attention to (cf. Leddy 2002).

Regarding Job and Wiesel, a reference was made of turning into liturgical forms of prayer. The cult has the task of representation (cf. Fuchs 2006; Fehling 2010), by making present, in securing the ritual, the reality which also applies "independently of experience" and is reality. It, so to speak, continues to "pray", although a person in their situation can possibly no longer pray (Franz 2000). In the ritual, mercy is present before the experience, also independent from it, in order to be experienced as such, in particular, as far as its pre-givenness is concerned.

The doxological liturgy becomes an area of idiosyncratic "sacramental" steadiness, namely the blessing to be told, in every case, and to experience that God (and hence hope) is always greater than happiness and the afflictions of humankind. The ritual is hence not only a condensed expression of human experience but is also opposed to the latter and represents a reality which can also be contrary to facts in respect to experience. What the ritual brings to attention is a promise which is, at present, not yet embedded, in many respects, in the experience of humans, but may be experienced with a view to hope, and often enough against all hope (cf. Rm 8, 24), as something which is nonetheless already in a certain way present reality.

The ritual represents the non-experienced, the outstanding. In the ritual, the God's answer occurs, now and in future rescuing, which is decided in God, and is hence genuine, but cannot yet be experienced. This applies, obviously, in particular to the ritual of anointing the critically ill or dying: in the face of the inevitability of death, there is belief in salvation from death.

Bibliography

Casper, Bernhard (1998): Das Ereignis des Betens. Grundlinien einer Hermeneutik des religiösen Geschehens, Freiburg/München: Alber.

Fehling, Ruth (2010): „Jesus ist für unsere Sünden gestorben". Eine praktisch-theologische Hermeneutik, Stuttgart: Kohlhammer.

Franz, Ansgar (2000) Klage als Ernstfall des Betens, in: U. Willers (Ed.), Beten: Sprache des Glaubens. Seele des Gottesdienstes, Tübingen: Francke, 435-475.

Fromm, Erich (1980): Ihr werdet sein wie Gott, Reinbek: Rowohlt.

Fuchs, Ottmar (1982): Die Klage als Gebet. Eine theologische Besinnung am Beispiel des Psalms 22, München: Kösel.

Fuchs, Ottmar (1987): Klage. Eine vergessene Gebetsform, in: H. Becker/B. Einig/ P.-O. Ullrich (Eds.), Im Angesicht des Todes: Ein interdisziplinäres Kompendium. St. Ottilien: EOS Verlag, 939-1024.

Fuchs, Ottmar (2001): Unerhörte Klage über den Tod hinaus! Überlegungen zur Eschatologie der Klage, in: M. Ebner (Ed.), Klage. Jahrbuch für Biblische Theologie, vol. 16, Neukirchen-Vluyn: Neuchkirchener Verlag.

Fuchs, Ottmar (2006): Aspekte einer praktischen Theologie der „Stellvertretung", in: J.C. Janowski/B. Janowski/H.P. Lichtenberger (Eds.), Stellvertretung. Theologische, philosophische und kulturelle Aspekte, Neukirchen-Vluyn: Neukirchener, 227-264.

Fuchs, Ottmar (2016): Der zerrissene Gott. Das trinitarische Gottesbild in den Brüchen der Welt, Ostfildern: Grünewald, vol. 3.

Fuchs, Ottmar (2017): Von der siegreichen Apologie zum verletzbaren Denken und Handeln, in: B. E. Koziel (Ed.), Apologie und Glaubensrechenschaft zwischen Konfrontation und Korrelation. Überlegungen zur Struktur gegenwärtiger Fundamentaltheologie. Würzburg: Echter, 383-403.

Fuchs, Ottmar (2018): Das Jüngste Gericht. Hoffnung über den Tod hinaus, Regensburg: Friedrich Pustet.

Hieke, Thomas (1998): Schweigen wäre gotteslästerlich, in: Bibel und Liturgie 71: 287-304.

Janowski, Bernd (2003): Konfliktgespräche mit Gott. Eine Anthropologie der Psalmen, Neukirchen-Vluyn: Neukirchener Verlag.

Leddy, Mary Jo (2002): Radical Gratitude, New York: Orbis Books.

Meier, Thomas M. (2012): Dürrenmatt und der Zufall, Ostfildern: Grünewald.

Müller, Augustinus R. (1996): Stimmungsumschwung im Klagepsalm, in: Archiv für Liturgiewissenschaft 28, 416-426.

Rahner, Karl (1980) Die unverbrauchbare Transzendenz Gottes und unsere Sorge um die Zukunft, in: K. Rahner, Schriften zur Theologie. Band 14, in Sorge um die Kirche. Zürich: Benziger, 405-421.

Schoors, Antoon (1984): Warum hast du mich verlassen? In: Geist und Leben 57, 3, 193-199.

Spiegel, Yorick (1973): Der Prozess des Trauerns, München: Kaiser 1973.

Steiof, Dorothee (2005): Das Gotteslob der Psalmen im Spannungsfeld von Macht und Gnade, in: R. Bucher/R. Krockauer (Ed.), Macht und Gnade, Münster: lit, 88-102.

Werbick, Jürgen (1996): Was das Beten der Theologie zu denken gibt, in: J.B. Metz/ J. Reigersdorfer/J. Werbick, Gottesrede, Münster: lit, 59-94.

Wiesel, Elie (1987): Der Prozess von Schamgorod, Freiburg i.Br.: Herder.

"Will you still need me …?"

Health Care Chaplaincy in the Face of Suffering

Jürgen Janik

This article explores the dimensions of suffering as they are encountered in the hospital setting. Various approaches of dealing with suffering in this context are presented. Asking for God, facing finiteness and imperfection mark the theological reflection. Finally, various dimensions of health care chaplaincy and its contribution to dealing with suffering are explicated.

The Experience of Suffering

Suffering becomes obvious in the hospital.

> I'm sick and lying down: I am on a different level, I no longer fully share the perspective of my environment. I look up, they look down at me… . I lie down, they stand. This is part of my loneliness as a sick person. The healthy talk to me, maybe they talk more about me. I am more argued about than a speaker. (Steffensky 1998, 11)[1]

Suffering is characterized by passivity and vulnerability. Loneliness and fear prevail. Suffering urges questions. The patient asks for the reason of the sickness, possible own fault or failure. "Does my suffering have a meaning? How can it be overcome?"

Some patients think about changing their way of life when they have overcome the illness. They newly reflect what is essential to life for them. Life is conceived to be negotiable. Patients want to regain the capacity to act and not to be powerless. For the patient suffering reveals (occasionally for the first time) the significance of a partnership and its capability to help bear the suffering. The immeasurable support of the partner is movingly realized. Relatives want to help, want to be active, and suffer themselves from not being able to help. They are "Co-Sufferers". Their unique role is to relieve the isolation of the patient.

In the hospital the patient suffers in three regards: from the illness, from the treatment of the illness and from the hospital treatment. Illness is

---

1 All translations here and below done by J. Janik.

experienced as insult to the sane and highly productive individual. The medical treatment with all its side effects is a blessing and a curse at the same time. It may cause further suffering. Physicians say, "first we make a person really sick (e.g. through chemotherapy), in order to cure them. This is hard to bear as success is not guaranteed." Patients suffer from the handling of their situation when they experience communication problems between medical disciplines. They feel they are "treated" rather than taken as respected partners in the handling of their sickness. Often they have to endure a long and ambiguous decision-making process before a palliative treatment is introduced. Patients from a migration background frequently do not feel well understood, not only because of the language barrier. "As far as illness and pain are concerned, both need to be understood not only on the bio-physical but also on the bio-cultural level." (Körtner 2009, 528) The different cultural or religious background and the understanding of illness that derives from it strains these patients and their families. Although they now live in a western individualized medical world, they still expect a family oriented and family based care and treatment.

Understanding Suffering and Dealing with Suffering

Suffering is an inevitable part of life.

> In paradise, Mother Teresa could not have developed into Mother Teresa … Only in a world of natural and moral evils can there be the peaks of human solidarity and altruistic devotion – values that we consider to be among human's highest possibilities and for which it is worth living. Even the Christian cardinal virtues of faith, hope and love only make sense in such a world. (Loichinger 2011, 6)

In their song "When I'm 64" the Beatles ask the crucial question "Will you still need me?" They do not only ask what someone needs to satisfy basic needs. Their challenging question is rather *who* needs me.

> The question is not directed at the person in need of help, but at others – including the helpers. This does not fit in with the usual division in the world of social services between service providers and recipients. The Beatles turn this everyday counterpart upside down: It is not the neediness of the old and frail person that is of interest, but its significance for others. (Mathwig 2014, 86)

Here, a change of paradigms is envisaged: The sufferers are of social relevance. As Johann Baptist Metz put it "Jesus' first glance did not aim at the sins of others but at the suffering of others" (Metz 1997, 200). He even claims an "authority of the sufferers" (Ibid., 202). We need the sufferers.

In the hospital, suffering serves as a "Scharnierbegriff" ("hinge term") (Moos et al. 2016, 197) for the different health care professionals that needs to be explicated in an individual situation. When the various professions share the experience of the suffering of a patient they are enabled to communicate beyond their professional boundaries and languages. Chaplains are agents of communication (Ibid., 195). Very often they facilitate the exchange between the professionals.

The "others" (i.e. medical and therapeutic professionals), have the active part. They are called for action and their vocabulary is that of struggle and fight while their aim is to cure or relieve suffering. This biophysical approach is successful in dealing with acute illnesses and pain. But in cases of chronic diseases a broader understanding of illness and health is needed, one that realizes that the whole person suffers from the illness physically, psychologically, socially and spiritually, and relatives and friends suffer as well (cf. Rumbold 2012, 178). Therefore the relational image of the human being needs to be taken into account. This leads to an understanding of relational autonomy rather than the notion of an idealized individualistic autonomy that neglects the vulnerable and dependent situation of the sick person.

The approach of salutogenesis developed by Aaron Antonovsky pinpoints the importance of the experience of coherence in dealing with suffering. Coherence has three components: the experience of *comprehensibility* that is evoked in the question "why do I have this illness"; the experience of *manageability* that refers the sick person to its individual resources and to ask for the support of others and for the help of "higher" or divine powers; and the experience of *meaningfulness* that refers the sick to his or her hitherto sustaining framework of the meaning of life and that motivates him/her to bear the actual suffering – even in naming its meaninglessness.

> But if a person can develop this threefold confidence that the events are:
> – understandable
> – influenceable
> – and are bound by meaning,
> the storms of life cannot harm him or her as much as people to whom events seem incomprehensible, uninfluenceable and meaningless. (Schneidereit-Mauth 2013, 413)

It is helpful to distinguish suffering from pain. Not every suffering is painful. Not every pain is experienced as suffering. For instance, the experience of pain in the course of a top-performing sports activity most likely is not experienced as suffering whereas somebody may suffer from her or his physical appearance although he/she is in good health.

> It is not only the length of time (e.g. chronic pain) that turns pain into suffering, but also the fact that pain becomes a threat at the level of existence, in other words, it questions the integrity of the person. (Schaupp 2017, 288)

Pain may be released or eased whereas suffering may be eased but not completely be taken away. The traditional works of bodily or mental mercy: visiting and comforting the sick, and consoling the grieving, are aimed not to take away the suffering but to bear it together to ease the suffering. Coming from a holistic approach, *spiritual suffering* also needs to be taken into account. Spiritual pain may be understood as "painful blank space" (Ibid., 290). One suffers from one's own incapability not to be able to follow an individually recognized meaning of life, or to have missed the truth of one's life, or to be culpable without having the chance of reconciliation, or to suffer from the discrepancy between one's own ideal and the reality of life.

> At the level of conscious existence, forms of pain and suffering emerge that are independent of somatic causes. They refer to what implicit ideas of salvation and wholeness we have of our life on a personal level, to values, relationships and goals that we experience as meaningful in a broad sense. (Ibid., 292)

The notion of spiritual suffering is not clearly defined. It very often comprises psychic pain, religious struggle and spiritual distress (Peng-Keller 2017, 295). This makes it obvious that the search for meaning and the quest for God are linked. Spiritual suffering influences the ability to cope with an illness and it needs to be addressed psychologically and spiritually.

The Theological Perspective: Asking for God, Facing Finiteness and Imperfection

"God whispers in our pleasures, speaks in our conscience, but shouts in our pain: it is His megaphone to rouse a deaf world" (Lewis 1940, 91). Various approaches offer the idea that the inexplicability of suffering is a part of the inexplicability of God (cf. Rahner 2010, 155); of divine solidarity and compassion of the "crucified God" (Moltmann 1972). "Our true suffering is his suffering as well, our sorrow is his sorrow, our pain is also the pain of his love." (Moltmann 1992, 781) Suffering is not explicable, but it is to be fought (Liberation Theology). In facing suffering, faith is speechless. The example of Job offers a theology of accusation, even rebellion. There are open questions that must be frankly posed to God.

> The biblical statements clearly testify that the disease has power over humans, but no rights to them. The power of sickness is also limited by the signs that announce the onset of God's dominion. That is why Jesus did not teach people to understand the meaning of their diseases, but healed them from their suffering in order to open them to the message of faith. (Schockenhoff 2013, 54)

There is a danger of religious interpretation of illness that it helps to integrate the illness in ones frame of life but for the sake of capitulation in front of the illness. If illness is simply seen as fate sent from God or as a way of purification or testing from God, this might lead to an obedient conformance with the illness, where resistance and struggle would be demanded. The reaction to suffering can not only be resignation, i.e. adaption to reality. The freedom of the person implies that humans are not only able to suffer. They are also able to hope. There is a dialectic between resistance and surrender to the irreversible (cf. Körtner 2009, 536).

> Also, the acceptance of a disease is a form of resistance; resistance to the fact that the disease dominates and paralyzes the whole person, plunges him/her into despair and a desperate and blind fight against the disease, which regards everything as "reparable" and all diseases and even death as abolishable. (Eibach 2009, 352)

Suffering confronts the limitations of life. In former times people suffered from fear of chaos. Today they suffer from the push to wholeness that is different from holiness. Faith and holiness believe in God's power to heal the broken, whereas the push to wholeness burdens the individual with the responsibility of bearing the brokenness and reestablishing wholeness by oneself. "A peculiar new suffering is emerging that burdens especially the most sensible: the suffering from not being perfect" (Steffensky 1998, 19). Health Care Chaplains are representatives of the limits and limitations of decisions, of treatments and of life. Chaplains dare to name limits and limitations and they invite to touch and transcend them. Health Care Chaplains resist the dictate of wholeness: the wholeness of understanding, of a good life, of good passing away; and finally, of the fixation on healthiness.

> Against the totalitarian terror, I would like to praise the successful half. The sweetness and beauty of life does not lie at the end, in perfect success and in wholeness. Life is finite, not only in the sense that we must die. The finiteness lies in life itself, in limited happiness, in limited things, in limited fullness. [...]
> One must be able to stop winning. One must be able to stop conquering the disease under all circumstances. There are diseases which belong to a person. But there is no disease that affects his/her dignity as a human being. (Ibid., 19f.)

So, the sick have a right to be sick. They are entitled to take refuge in the hospital, in their room, in their bed. They have a right to be impaired or disabled.

Health Care Chaplaincy: the Anthropological and the Structural Role

Health Care Chaplaincy is teamwork. All caregiving of the various health professions presupposes the awareness of the caregiver's capacity to suffer, to be vulnerable, to be bound to temporality and to be mortal. Caregivers need to be prepared to endure despair and fear and to be touchable. They also endure the inexplicability and meaninglessness of the suffering and are often tongue-tied. Health Care Chaplains – similar to other health Care professionals – share an anthropologically symbolic role.

> The experts do not only stand for treatment, but also for being caught with suffering. They are also representatives of humanity ... Their roles are related to central human values: to health, to physical and mental integrity, but also to care when one cannot (any longer) help oneself. (Weiher 2014a, 121)

Health Care Professionals value the sick in their personhood, and their experience of dignity. "Such experience of dignity remains even when the caregiver leaves." (Weiher 2014b, 419) Dealing with suffering is part of their professional self-understanding. In desperate moments all caregivers may adopt the task of surrogate hope for the sick person by inviting the patient to leave the hope for recovery to the proceedings of the health care institution and professional treatment (cf. Weiher 2014a, 175).

Health Care Chaplains want to help bear, and at best to reduce, the suffering from the harm caused by the illness. They are advocates for the patient within the system and occasionally in confronting the health system. They cooperate in the structures of clinical ethics consultation and other forms of clinical consultation. Health Care Chaplaincy has to deal with questions about the ethics of the conduct of life, questions about decision making concerning treatment, and questions about the ethics of the health care institution and its culture. These are dealt with in structured and non-structured formats. In this context the chaplain needs to develop an ethical "meta competence" (Moos et al. 2016, 298) that involves dealing with morals, their ethical role as chaplain and their own professional ethos. Insofar, health care chaplaincy becomes "lived ethics".

Health Care Chaplains Provide Spiritual Care

Awareness for the afflicted person to empower him/her to face the individual situation, and to deal with it in a constructive beneficial way, is essential. The instruments of health care chaplaincy are: being present, being in dialogue and providing rituals. Being present: having time for patients, relatives and professionals is a precious resource of Health Care Chaplaincy; "having time" appears paradoxically in the haste of the clinical setting; being present embraces the situation of the counterpart in its wholeness and complexity without being focused only on the illness. Dialogue involves listening, being silent, interpreting and witnessing. Ritual can help process a situation in prayer, sacrament and blessing, and to connect it with the faith community.

Health Care Chaplains keep silence and bear witness – also that God is missed. For them silence is an ethical attitude. A physician cannot keep silent. His/her scheme is anamnesis, diagnosis and therapy. Chaplains allow themselves to be touched by the suffering of the person and abstain from presenting any draft standard. They cannot explain God. "I do not know" frees them from phrases of consolation and faith that fail to have substance. One will not understand everything and one does not need to do so.

> Communication of the gospel means enduring heartbreak. To endure non-knowing and non-understanding. It also means to weigh faith. Yet to hope, to empathize, to love; to contradict the dark, not to give it the last word; to miss God, to seek God and to assert God – and thus the truth of mercy, justice and reverence for life. (Brems 2016, 538)

Health Care Chaplaincy aims to broaden the perspective of patients by making their individual spirituality accessible to them as a resource to cope with their situation (Weiher 2014). Spirituality is conceived of two perspectives: a broad existential and implicit sense as thread of one's life, as search for meaning, for oneself, for holism and as an explicit transcendent perspective of connectedness with the divine, the sacred or a higher power (cf. Schaupp 2017, 289). Both approaches cannot be separated since a transcendent meaning is mostly encoded in existential experiences.

> Spirituality is a person's (conscious and unconscious) potential in self and world sensations, in experiences of meaning and the creation of meaning as well as in attitudes and attitudes towards life. Out of this potential, life, person, and world receive meaning and people give meaning to themselves and life. (Weiher 2017, 22)

Furthermore, Christian spirituality is an outcry. It has an option for the needy and deprived and it points to the ultimately deprived crucified savior, Jesus

Christ. It calls for conversion and transformation on the individual and the social and institutional level.

In times of suffering belief has different coping capacities. It can be affirmative, negating, critical and/or transformative. If faith functions affirmative, belief is experienced as a foothold. In this situation Health Care Chaplains are asked to help patients to hold on to their faith practice, or to help to restore a former religious practice that helps to deal with the illness. Occasionally patients actively question or negate faith in God when the closeness and help of God is not felt. This may result in turning away the visit of the chaplain, or, more beneficially in a critical reflection about the image of God one has or one has been taught to have. The search for God may be or become the form of believing (desiderium desiderii). Some patients take the experience of their illness as a task to grow in life. They say, "I asked myself why not me?" and in doing so, they provide a meaning for their suffering. This transformative approach strives to integrate suffering as an inevitable part of life. Such inner overcoming can help to accept the limitation of life and frees one from false expectations towards life. It may allow to adopt an attitude of serenity and indifference that lead to the insight that chronic disease and long suffering do not make life absurd and undignified (cf. Schockenhoff 2013, 54f.).

Health Care Chaplaincy: the Helper is the Help

Health Care Chaplains bring awareness that suffering has a reverse side that is intense relatedness, love, and the experience of mutual endurance of severe situations; "The essential help is – above all deed – the helper." (Splett 1996, 220) Health Care Chaplains, being reliable to the patient, perform something like "embodied consolation". Consolation happens in contact and relation. It is less a verbal activity than a form of reliable presence.

> A central moment of consolation is to let the other suffer. The suffering is not talked away, it is not negated by gestures or rites, but it is respected, appreciated, taken seriously, felt. It is precisely this "letting happen" that makes it possible for suffering and the suffering person to change – in suffering, not outside suffering. (Aurnhammer 2011, 61)

Compassion is not regretting, but showing solidarity in staying with the suffering as a helpful counterpart. This implies respect for the otherness of the suffering person and his/her worldview, their adherence to another religion or their being non-religious. Empathetic reliability is a basic ethical attitude of health care chaplains. Even without words, but through a gaze or a gesture, the sick and vulnerable person is dignified. Hereby the Health Care Chaplain implicitly or explicitly symbolizes divine accompaniment and compassion.

Finally, Health Care Chaplaincy invites one to take the perspective of "another wholeness" that is not afraid of suffering and where everything is in good hands. We need the sufferers. Saying this neither justifies suffering nor (even worse) exploits suffering. Rather, this approach enforces the need for compassionate communities that integrate those who suffer, are frail or impaired.

Bibliography

Aurnhammer, Klaus (2011): Jenseits von Verkündigung. Religion und Trost in der Postmoderne, in: Leidfaden. Fachmagazin für Krisen, Leid und Trauer 0: 60-70. Online: https://s3-eu-central-1.amazonaws.com/nbz-ncc-vur/media/pdf/17/06/53/Probeheft_Leidfaden_0_2011.pdf (last access 03/13/2019).

Brems, Michael (2016): Flügel Liebe Ruh. Krankenhausseelsorge als Ort religiöser Erfahrung, in: Wege zum Menschen 68, 6: 529-540. Online: https://doi.org/10.13109/weme.2016.68.6.529 (last access 03/13/2019).

Eibach, Ulrich (2009): Umgang mit schwerer Krankheit. Widerstand, Ergebung, Annahme, in: G. Thomas/I. Karle (Eds.): Krankheitsdeutung in der postsäkularen Gesellschaft. Stuttgart: Kohlhammer, 339-353.

Körtner, Ulrich H.J. (2009): Leiden – Grenzen des Verstehens, in: G. Thomas/I. Karle (Eds.): Krankheitsdeutung in der postsäkularen Gesellschaft. Stuttgart: Kohlhammer, 526-542.

Lewis, Clive S. (1940): The Problem of Pain, New York: Harper/Collins.

Loichinger, Alexander (2011): Die Frage nach Gott angesichts menschlichen Leids, in: Religionsunterricht heute 39, 1: 4-8. Online: http://downloads.bistummainz.de/5/455/1/40935408114320660751.pdf (last access 03/13/2019).

Mathwig, Frank (2014): "Will you still need me, will you still feed me … ?" Bedeutung haben – auch in Krankheit und Sterben, in: I. Noth/C. Kohli Reichenbach (Eds.): Palliative und Spiritual Care. Aktuelle Perspektiven in Medizin und Theologie. Zürich: Theologischer Verlag Zürich, 85-101.

Metz, Johann Baptist (1997): Im Pluralismus der Religions- und Kulturwelten. Anmerkungen zu einem theologisch-politischen Weltprogramm, in: J. B. Metz: Zum Begriff der neuen Politischen Theologie 1967-1997. Mainz: Matthias-Grünewald-Verlag, 197-206.

Moltmann, Jürgen (1972): Der gekreuzigte Gott, München: Christian Kaiser Verlag.

Moltmann, Jürgen (1992): Leiden, in: C. Schütz (Ed.): Praktisches Lexikon der Spiritualität. Freiburg: Herder, 775-782.

Moos, Thorsten/Ehm, Simone/Kliesch, Fabian/Thiesbonenkamp-Maag, Julia (2016): Ethik in der Klinikseelsorge, Göttingen: Vandenhoeck & Ruprecht.

Peng-Keller, Simon (2017): Spiritual Pain. Annäherung an einen Schlüsselbegriff inter-professioneller Spiritual Care, in: Spiritual Care 6, 3: 295-302. Online: https://www.degruyter.com/downloadpdf/j/spircare.2017.6.issue-3/spircare-2016-0207/spircare-2016-0207.pdf (last access 03/13/2019).

Rahner, Karl (2010): Warum lässt uns Gott leiden?, in: A. Loichinger/A. Kreiner (Eds.), Theodizee in den Weltreligionen. Ein Studienbuch. Paderborn: UTB, 146-157.

Rumbold, Bruce (2012): Models of spiritual care, in: M. Cobb/C.M. Puchalski/B. Rumbold (Eds.): Oxford textbook of spiritualty in healthcare. New York: Oxford, 177-183.

Schaupp, Walter (2017): Die spirituelle Dimension des Schmerzes, in: Spiritual Care 6, 3: 285-293.

Schneidereit-Mauth, Heike (2013): Spiritualität als heilsame Kraft. Ein Plädoyer für Spiritual Care in der Klinik, in: Wege zum Menschen 65, 5: 404-418. Online: https://doi.org/10.13109/weme.2013.65.5.404 (last access 03/13/2019).

Schockenhoff, Eberhard (2013): Die religiöse Deutung der Krankheit, in: Spiritual Care 2, 3: 49-56.

Splett, Jörg (1996): Schmerz und Leid als Konturen der Freiheit. Gedanken christlicher Anthropologie, in: Zeitschrift für medizinische Ethik 42: 217-232.

Steffensky, Fulbert (1998): Wie gehen wir mit dem Leid um? Wie geht das Leid mit uns um?, in: G. Adam/R. Kollmann/A. Pithan (Eds.): Mit Leid umge-hen. Dokumentationsband des sechsten Würzburger religionspädagogischen Symposiums. Münster: Comenius-Institut, 11-21.

Weiher, Erhard (2014a): Das Geheimnis des Lebens berühren – Spiritualität bei Krankheit, Sterben, Tod, 4th ed., Stuttgart: Kohlhammer.

Weiher, Erhard (2014b): Spiritualität und Würdeempfinden. Möglichkeiten spiritu-eller Begleitung am Lebensende, in: N. Feinendegen/G. Höver/A. Schaeffer/K. Westerhorstmann (Eds.): Menschliche Würde und Spiritualität in der Begleitung am Lebensende. Impulse aus Theorie und Praxis. Würzburg: Königshausen & Neumann, 411-424.

Weiher, Erhard (2017): Symbolische Kommunikation in Seelsorge und Spiritual Care, in: S. Peng-Keller (Ed.): Bilder als Vertrauensbrücken. Die Symbolsprache Sterbender verstehen. Berlin: de Gruyter, 17-34.

Humanist Approaches to Spiritual Care in Patient Counseling in the Netherlands

Carlo Leget

In most Western countries, health care chaplaincy is organized by religious institutions. The large majority of chaplains are ordained Christian ministers who are employed by the church. Their response to suffering is inspired by their own religious tradition. Although they are open to people from other traditions, and proselytizing is seen as an unethical way of dealing with vulnerable patients, their spiritual counseling is based on a religious worldview.

In this contribution, we will focus on a country and a practice, which is largely nonreligious. In the Netherlands, the majority of patients do not believe in a personal God and are not affiliated with any religious tradition. Do these people receive spiritual counseling, and if so, what does it look like? Is it possible to offer spiritual counseling without a religious background?

In order to answer these questions, we will first provide some more information about non-believers in the Netherlands. Subsequently, we will focus on one specific tradition: humanist spiritual counseling. In order to give a concrete example of what non-religious counseling looks like, we will define and develop a model for spiritual counseling of patients receiving palliative care, their families and their caregivers.

Humanism in the Netherlands

According to a survey done approximately every 10 years over the last half-century, in 2015 only 14% of the Dutch population believed in a personal God. In 1966 47% of the population still considered themselves theists. This number gradually dropped in the subsequent decades to 28% who consider themselves so called "ietsisten" (people who believe in "iets" [something], by which they mean an undefined higher power); 34% who consider themselves agnostic; and 24% of the population who consider themselves atheists (Bernts/Berghuis 2016).

If we look at the spiritual landscape of the Netherlands from a different perspective, focusing on people who consider themselves non-religious, according to another source the landscape looks a bit different. According to the

© BRILL SCHÖNINGH, 2022 | DOI:10.30965/9783657715428_016

report of the Scientific Council of the Government from 2006 entitled "Belief in the public domain", 18% of Dutch people consider themselves non-religious and non-humanistic; 16% consider themselves non-religious and moderately humanistic; 12% consider themselves humanistic; and 26% see themselves as non-denominational spiritual (van de Donk et al. 2006).

The problem with figures like these, of course, is the way the different categories are defined, the way these definitions are perceived by the respondents, and the question of whether people would have given different answers if they had been approached in a different way. In the field of spirituality and religion especially, words are defined in a great many ways, sometimes even contradictory ways, as is seen in the many definitions there are of the very concepts of spirituality and religion themselves. We do not know how words are interpreted in the minds of respondents from a variety of cultural backgrounds, even in one country.

In this contribution, the focus will be on one specific tradition of a life philosophy outside of religious traditions in the Netherlands: humanism. The Humanist Association was founded in February 1946, as a reaction against the atrocities that had taken place in World War II. The co-founder and spiritual father of this organization was Jaap van Praag (1911-1981), a man of Jewish origin who had survived the Second World War by going underground. During the time that he hid, he reflected on the question of what would be needed to rebuild Europe in such a way that a war like that could not happen again. He dreamt of a civilization of respect and tolerance built on a shared humanity. In order to achieve this goal, he identified two battles. The first battle (in his words the "minor battle"), was against the domination of Christianity and religious dogma in society. The second battle (the "major battle"), was against nihilism and for the promotion of spiritual resilience (Derkx 2004).

As early as the 1950s, Jaap van Praag wrote about humanist spiritual counseling, which he considered to be an important service to non-religious people. In 1962, the Humanist Association created an education program for spiritual counselors in the military. In 1964, the Humanist Education Institute was founded for the education of spiritual counselors. In 1989, this Institute became the University of Humanistic Studies, a university providing a six year program for the education of humanist chaplains working in all sectors of society.

The Humanist Association houses people of different views, convictions and backgrounds. Some agree with van Praag that the major battle of our culture is against nihilism and for the promotion of spiritual resilience, which can be inspired by both religious or non-religious traditions. For others the major battle is against all forms of religion, promoting a militant atheism in which there is no place for any type of religion. Although in many countries human-ism is defined by being non-religious, in the Netherlands many of humanists are open to spiritual or religious elements.

According to Peter Derkx, professor of humanism at the University of Humanistic Studies until 2017, two principles may function as a shared core of the many varieties of Humanism: 1) the view that every philosophy of life ("levensbeschouwing") is contextual and constructed by humans; and 2) the conviction that all people are equal and should be treated equally, because the unique value and irreplaceability of every individual are essential elements of humanism (Derkx 2011). Given these two tenets, what does humanism look like in regard to its content as a philosophy of life? And what does this mean for spiritual counseling?

Humanist Spiritual Counseling

According to Ninian Smart, worldviews or life philosophies can be divided into seven dimensions that, taken together, form a whole, which helps people ori-ent their lives (Smart 1989). When we consider the humanist tradition through this lens the following picture appears (Alma/Anbeek 2011).

Dimensions of Humanism

As for the narrative and mythical dimension, there are many stories expressing the humanity of human beings, which are considered important, stemming from a great number of backgrounds. There are, however, no holy books or a specific canon, which separate humanists from non-humanists. More impor-tant than defining which texts are of value and which are not, is the great importance attached to hermeneutics. Because of the fact that all narratives are seen as contextual and reflecting human experiences, the interpretation of texts is an hermeneutical enterprise in which many layers and voices can be discerned. As little as texts are univocal, human beings themselves are seen as such. Humanists see the self as a dialogical self, and an important goal of humanist counseling is aimed at listening to the inner dialogues of this self (Hermans/Kempen 1993).

The doctrinal and philosophical dimension of humanism is characterized by a never ending dialogue between different systematic articulations of what humanism is. This never ending dialogue precludes a humanist doctrine, apart from the shared basis identified by Peter Derkx. Humanists are anti-dogmatic, sometimes even to the paradox of proclaiming this anti-dogmatism as a dogma, and value critical reflection above all answers.

According to the ethical and legal dimension of humanism, a balance is sought between individual well-being and contribution to a humane society. In the work of Jaap van Praag there was already a balance between the individual and the community, which were seen as both important, not sacrificing one for the other. As for personal ethics much effort has been given in recent years by ethics professor Joep Dohmen to develop an art of living based on authors like Michel Foucault and Pierre Hadot, comparable to the work of Wilhelm Schmid in Germany.

The ritual dimension of the humanist tradition is perhaps the one which is least developed. Humanists do not have a tradition of rituals they can fall back upon. Nevertheless, since 2017 the University of Humanist Studies has offered a course for ritual accompaniment of life events, called a celebrant education.

As for the emotional and experiential dimension of humanism, there is no such thing as revelation or authority outside of humanity. All knowledge which is acknowledged is based on human experience. Among humanists there may, however, be disagreement about the openness to interpretations of the source of these experiences, which is reflected in people belonging to inclusive or exclusive (atheistic) forms of humanism.

The social and institutional dimension of humanism is characterized by loose structures and small numbers. The Humanist Association in the Netherlands has about 17.000 members. Because humanism seems to be attractive to people who are critical of traditions, rules and organizational structures, it is hard to estimate how many people outside of the Humanist Association can be considered humanists. Nevertheless, besides the national organizations, there has also been an International Humanist and Ethical Union since 1952.

As for the material dimension of the humanist worldview, there are no specific devotion places or objects. If anything in this dimension has to be mentioned, it is the great works of art that reflect the greatness and vulnerability of humanity. Places of remembrance can have a similar value, as they document the value of humanity.

Competencies for Humanist Spiritual Counseling

Having sketched out the seven dimensions of humanism as a worldview, which may help people outside religious traditions to deal with life contingencies, what does humanist spiritual counseling look like? Hans Alma and Christa Anbeek describe their view on humanist counselling, building on Kenneth Pargament's finding that in crisis people tend to hold on to the way people have found meaning in their lives (Alma/Anbeek 2011). Spiritual counselors help people articulate the (broken) stories of their lives. By listening, they help collect fragments of what is important to them. A first step in this process is being open to whatever the patients tell them, and respecting their pain. The second step is an emotional experience of wonder or connectedness. What core competencies are needed to provide this form of spiritual counseling?

First, a hermeneutic competence is needed. Counselors should be able to read the existential meaning of human experiences and have the capacity to start a dialogue about this dimension. It may be necessary to have some specific knowledge about the religious or spiritual background of the patient, in order to understand what is at stake for this individual. For a genuine dialogue, however, it is also important to know one's own humanistic background, and one needs dialogical competencies and the ability to switch between sources and experiences.

Second, a self-reflective competency is needed. Humanist spiritual counseling is not a neutral technique, which can be separated from the person of the counsellor. It is this inner dialogue of the spiritual counsellor, which helps develop a spiritual or existential identity that plays an important role in the dialogue. Because the dialogue is between two unique human beings bringing their own existential identity to the conversation it may have a certain quality and intensity based on a shared humanity. In this intrapersonal and interpersonal dialogue the humanistic tradition may function as a "collective voice" (Hermans/Kempen 1993).

The third core competency needed can be called a heuristic competence based on an attitude of not knowing, a readiness to go on searching in the spiritual landscape of the patient. The goal of this process is not repairing the course of the old river, but supporting new currents that make the spiritual landscape of the conversation partner fertile again.

Example: a New Art of Dying

Since the 1960s the Dutch have developed a different response to end-of-life suffering than other countries in north Western Europe have. After a number of medical ethical discussions in the 1960s and 1970s, since the 1980s a growing number of Dutch citizens felt that there were no fundamental objections to a practice in which patients could have medical assistance in dying. After comprehensive national surveys among physicians in the 1990s, in 2001, a law was passed to allow euthanasia and physician-assisted dying under a number of preconditions. In 2002 the law went into effect (Onwuteaka-Philipsen et al. 2012).

The 50 years during which the euthanasia act was being prepared and developed coincided with the same period of time during which the religious landscape eroded and changed into a secularized society. Although it is tempting to see a direct correlation between the decrease of the influence of religion and the increase of euthanasia proponents, the relation between the two developments is more complex (Leget 2017a). The plea for euthanasia was also supported by members of Christian churches, at the same time as Western culture experienced the rise of neoliberalism according to which worldviews and religiousness were seen as a private matter. Parallel to the rise of neoliberalism, medical science developed into more and more specialties and a medicalization of many areas of life took place, including the beginning and end of life.

The art of dying model presented here has its origins in the research done in two nursing homes in Rotterdam between 1998-1999 (Leget 2017b). Although both nursing homes were part of an umbrella organization with a Roman Catholic background, it was striking that there was hardly any common framework to address spiritual issues and empower patients and proxies. Because a common framework and language was lacking, it was also difficult to integrate spiritual care in the interdisciplinary approach, which is characteristic of palliative care. The goal of developing a contemporary art of dying was to develop such a contemporary framework for spiritual issues, open to people from both religious and non-religious traditions, and meant to be used as a tool for conversation and reflection.

The first question is where to start and how to find a shared idea of what the goal of spiritual care is, and how the criteria of good spiritual care can be defined. In the context of a specific worldview or religious tradition, this question can be answered by referring to that tradition. But how to answer it from a non-denominational perspective? Would patient satisfaction be a good outcome? From a spiritual point of view, patient satisfaction may be a weak indicator of spiritual development, for spiritual struggles can be long, hard and not exactly satisfying at first sight. How does one solve this problem?

Inner Space

In order to develop a non-denominational framework for spiritual counselling at the end of life, empirical research was started in two nursing homes, resulting in the retrieval of a medieval tradition that had been helpful for a number of centuries (Leget 2007). During observation in the palliative wards of the nursing homes, one observation was that some health care professionals were continuously looking for what they called "space" for emotional processes to take place, problems to be solved, or family members to meet. Focusing on this idea of space as something in and between people, the idea was developed that perhaps here we could have a low profile entry to spiritual care which is accessible to every human being, whatever his or her cultural or (non)religious background is.

A conversation between a physician and an older female patient who asked about the possibility of euthanasia without having any idea of alternative options demonstrates how the idea of space might work in practice (Ibid.). At the beginning of the conversation, the patient spoke from fear and with a demanding tone. She wanted to be sure that there would be a way out of her suffering, a last escape in the form of euthanasia, if the pain became unbearable. At that time, the possibility of euthanasia had not been put into legislation yet, and the nursing home where the conversation took place was a Roman Catholic organization, not open to euthanasia. A dilemma seemed to arise, an impossible choice between the final wishes of the patient on the one hand, and the options and convictions of the palliative care physician on the other. As the physician listened with an open mind and open heart, however, the atmosphere in the room changed, and an honest conversation took place in which the patient felt acknowledged and the physician expressed her commitment to be available for the patient. Addressing the question at a different level, the underlying fear of an unknown dark future, and investing in the relationship between physician and patient, the dilemma was resolved in an unexpected way.

Reflecting on this conversation, it became clear that the quality of this conversation was made possible by the amount of openness and inner freedom the physician displayed. Metaphorically, this could be called "inner space". The inner space of the physician enabled her to express her emotions, and by being heard the patient in her turn developed inner space. This process of exchange seemed to be a promising point of departure for a practice of spiritual care which is not based on any denominational framework, but on a shared humanity.

Beyond Relativism

Taking inner space as the starting point and goal of spiritual care may sound like a relativist position. It could be so if inner space were seen as an emotion of feeling indifferent about something or someone, similar to a stoic *apatheia* in which nothing really matters. Inner space as it is developed in the *ars moriendi* model, however, is not an emotion but a metaphor for a state of mind. This state of mind is characterized by openness and the ability to experience a variety of thoughts and feelings simultaneously. The physician in the story might simultaneously feel compassion for the patient in view of her fears about her future, aversion to the demanding tone of the patient, surprise about how little the patient knows about palliative care options, and sympathy for the strength she displays by asking for help in dying. Inner space is a state of mind which enables people to experience all these things, without being swept away or influenced by one of them. It allows one to open up to one's inner polyphony, and discover how every one of these voices may lead to the moral and spiritual good that is sought.

As a way to open up to one's inner polyphony, inner space is important to both partners in a conversation. By being attuned to the inner space of the patient, the physician becomes attuned to the inner freedom of the patient, as the starting point of morality. As long as the thoughts and feelings of this patient are motivated by fear, there is a lack of inner freedom, and any moral choice is compromised. Focusing on inner space helps to retrieve the inner freedom needed to make moral choices and enable spiritual growth. This is not a cognitive or rational process, although cognition and rationality are part of the spiritual process. Inner space can be sensed and felt on the level of humanity as embodied by the patient. As rational animals, we sense when people have inner freedom to a lesser or greater degree. Inner space is a universally shared human experience when we are relaxed and joyful; it enhances creativity and the discovery of new horizons and solutions. The metaphor as such is of a formal nature, not attached to any specific religious or spiritual tradition, and is at the crossroads of psychology, spirituality, ethics, philosophy and theology. Some people want to make it more concrete by connecting it with mindfulness, others see a relationship with the bracketing we know from phenomenology; the openness of the metaphor allows for more than one way of working with it.

By taking inner space as the starting point and goal of spiritual care, and by claiming that inner space is a metaphor referring to a state of mind which is more or less of a formal nature, namely, enabling listening to one's inner polyphony, the question remains what the content of the moral and spiritual process is. In the *ars moriendi* model this question is not directly answered, but postponed, by virtue of its openness to different spiritual traditions. In order to explain how this works, we have to explain the second component of the *ars moriendi* model: the retrieval of a medieval tradition.

Retrieving the Ars Moriendi Tradition

At the end of the middle ages, the Black Plague caused the death of millions of people within a few years, causing one of the great collective traumas of the West. As a response to this situation small block books appeared with both pictures and texts in order to prepare people for a good death. The dying process was depicted as a spiritual struggle of the dying person, surrounded by devils testing the virtues of hope, faith, charity, patience and humility on the one hand, and angels supporting the dying person in the recovery of these virtues on the other. The texts can be read as an expression of the inner polyphony of the dying: the spiritual struggle externalized in the struggle between demons and angels (Bayard 1999; Girard-Augry 1986).

The contemporary art of dying model is inspired by its medieval predecessor, with three fundamental changes. First, the five virtues and vices are replaced by their underlying anthropological themes. Second, the binary between good and bad is replaced by a continuum according to which the two poles of the opposition are both seen as morally neutral and of equal importance. Third, the character of choice (either virtue or vice) is replaced by an acceptance of the inner polyphony, in which people can have opposing feelings and thoughts simultaneously.

The first theme of the *ars moriendi* model concerns the question "Who am I and what do I really want?" The central theme of (patient) autonomy is placed within the opposition of being connected with oneself and being connected with others, in accordance with a philosophy of the self as developed by the French philosopher Paul Ricœur (Ricœur 1990). In the *ars moriendi* model the question of autonomy is reframed as the question of having inner space of discerning the different ways in which one is more or less attached to both oneself and the others, and asking oneself what would bring the inner freedom to discover the moral and spiritual good.

The second theme of the model is about the question "How do I deal with suffering?" This question is investigated against the background of the universal theme of doing and undergoing. In a culture focusing on interventions, outcomes and problem-solving, one needs inner space to reflect on the question of whether our choices are really free or part of a social and professional context which limits our ability to deal with suffering.

The third theme of the model revolves around the question "How can I say goodbye?" and involves the tension between holding on and letting go. Again, these two are placed on a continuum which helps reveal one's own inner space and is open to an integration of both extremes: As we know from bereavement studies, for example, letting go might not so much mean cutting bonds, but holding on to the beloved departed in a different way (Klass et al. 2014).

The fourth question is "How do I look back on my life?" In the tension between remembering and forgetting people may find or lose inner space when they are confronted with guilt, shame, gratefulness, and questions of forgiveness and reconciliation. Both extremes might be simultaneously there, or even integrated as in forgiveness in which there is an act of remembering ("bringing into the present") and forgetting ("changing the meaning it had in the past") at the same time.

The fifth question "What can I hope for?" is placed on the continuum between knowing and believing. Both scientific knowledge on the one hand and dogmatic belief on the other, may be a great source of security, but what happens to the openness and inner freedom of the person trying to make sense of what is happening? Again, inner space is an important state of mind in a culture in which spirituality and religion are subjectivized and privatized. Finding one's own way in these matters asks for a process of dialogue in which both partners authentically search outward from their inner space.

Working with the Model

The *ars moriendi* model can be used in a number of ways. As we have seen in some of the themes, it can be applied to both the level of contemporary culture in general and the intra- or interpersonal level (Leget 2016). In the Netherlands and Belgium, the model is used as a framework for reflection for patients who are admitted to the hospital and their families. It is used in the spiritual care training of all kinds of health care professionals in order to emphasize the importance of moving from the inner space outward which is available, and helping them to organize themes. It is used for spiritual history taking by health care professionals (nurses, physicians) who have had brief training in spiritual care; some chaplains use it for spiritual assessment in order to look at the inner space of the patient or discover their own blind spots in conversations. It is also used for reporting in patient files and transfer to hospice, in nursing homes and hospital wards (Leget 2017b).

Because the model is abstract with openness, it can be used in many ways. But what about the normative side of it? If the inner space is both the starting point and the goal of spiritual care, and the five themes and the tensions of the *ars moriendi* model only help discover the inner polyphony and dimensions of the themes, can it help to find out what is morally right and wrong? As the model is based on a shared humanity, it can only help define a space of conversation and encounter. It is the specific contextually mediated identity of the conversation partners who, with the model, determine what process takes place and what outcome is found. People working from a particular Christian background may work with the model and reframe the basic anthropological themes from a particular Christian perspective (Ibid.). The fact that the common anthropological basis is clarified may help to build a bridge between the conversation partners, and help them zoom out to seek a shared horizon. Putting so much emphasis upon enabling a conversation in which one's inner freedom can be discovered against the background of one's inner polyphony instead of giving moral directions is a big difference between the medieval version of the model and its contemporary version. At the same time, it expresses

an ethical choice putting the quality of the process of discovering inner freedom and responsibility above the outcome of the process. That brings us back
to the competencies of the professionals working with the model, in our case
the humanist chaplain.

The Humanist Core Competencies Revisited

As the three core competencies for humanist spiritual counseling interact, the
order in which they are discussed is more or less irrelevant. Departing from
the metaphor of inner space, a striking similarity can be observed with heuristic competence, which is characterized by an attitude of not knowing and
a readiness to continue searching for answers. Just as inner space is related to
the creativity and freshness of human consciousness, humanism relies on the
ability of human beings to find new horizons of meaning.

The self-reflective competence of the spiritual counselor, in which he/she
also relates to the polyphony of one's intra- and interpersonal dialogues, helps
to discover and maintain one's own inner space. It is here that the content of
the humanist tradition may be integrated as a consciously appropriated part of
an authentic and practiced philosophy of life. This gives access to the sources
of the spiritual tradition(s) one relates to.

Last, the hermeneutic competence, is important for discerning the existential meaning of the experiences which are discussed in the conversation, and
being able to relate this to the spiritual framework of both oneself and the
patient. Inner space is also needed for creative interpretation and the weighing of different possibilities. The five tensions of the *ars moriendi* model may
be helpful as an anthropological framework pointing to the shared humanity
connecting both conversation partners.

Bibliography

Alma, Hans/Anbeek, Christa (2011): Humanistisch levensbeschouwen en interlevens-
    beschouwelijke geestelijke verzorging, in: Tijdschift voor Humanistiek 46, 12: 68-77.
Bayard, Florence (1999): L'art du bien mourir au XVe siècle, Paris: Presses de l'Université
    Paris-Sorbonne.
Bernts, Ton/Berghuijs, Joantine (2016): God in Nederland 2006-2015, Utrecht: Ten Have.
Derkx, Peter (2004): Om de geestelijke weerbaarheid van humanisten: Teksten van
    Jaap van Praag, Utrecht: Humanistisch archief.
Derkx, Peter (2011): Humanisme, zinvol leven en nooit meer "ouder worden", Brussel:
    VUB Press.

Girard-Augry, Pierre (1986): Ars moriendi (1492) ou L'art de bien mourir. Paris: Dervy.

Hermans, Hubert/Kempen, Harry (1993): The dialogical self. Meaning as movement. San Diego: Academic Press.

Klass, Dennis/Silverman, Phyllis R./Nickman, Steven L. (Eds.) (2014): Continuing bonds. New understandings of grief, Philadelphia: Taylor & Francis.

Leget, Carlo (2007): Retrieving the Ars moriendi tradition, in: Medicine Health Care & Philosophy 10: 313-319.

Leget, Carlo (2016): A new art of dying as a cultural challenge, in: Studies in Christian Ethics, 29, 3: 279-285.

Leget, Carlo (2017a): The relation between cultural values, euthanasia, and spiritual care in the Netherlands, in: Polish archives of internal medicine 127, 4: 261-266.

Leget, Carlo (2017b): Art of living, art of dying. Spiritual care for a good death. London and Philadelphia: Jessica Kingsley Publishers.

Onwuteaka-Philipsen, Bregje/Brinkman-Stoppelenburg, Arianne/Penning, Corine/ de Jong-Krul, Gwen/van Delden, Johannes/van der Heide, Agnes (2012) Trends in end-of-life practices before and after the enactment of the euthanasia law in the Netherlands from 1990 to 2010. A repeated cross-sectional survey, in: Lancet 380: 908-915.

Ricœur, Paul (1990): Soi-même comme un autre, Paris: Seuil.

Smart, Ninian (1989): The world's religions, Cambridge: Cambridge University Press.

Van de Donk, W.B.H.J./Jonkers, A.P./Kronjee, G.J./Plum, R.J.J.M. (Eds.) (2006): Geloven in het publieke domein. Verkenning van een dubbele transformatie, Amsterdam: University Press.

Psychological and Psychotherapeutic Counseling of Palliative Care Patients

Urs Münch

Introduction

Psychologists as well as social workers and hospital chaplains have to offer vital support to help relieve the suffering of patients in palliative care, and provide support for their loved ones. However, psychologists are still not established throughout all settings: in hospitals, psychological support only needs to be provided if a palliative care unit wants to obtain a certain certificate. Outside hospital care, it is even more difficult to get psychologists involved in palliative care (Gramm/Münch 2017, 33f.; Münch/Gramm/Berthold 2016, 82). This leads to the strange situation that psychologists hardly contribute their knowledge to palliative care, although they are supposed to be specialists in at least one of the four dimensions of palliative care: physical, psychological, social and spiritual.

All four dimensions of palliative care overlap in some areas, so that the fields of social care, psychological care and spiritual care have many topics in common. Therefore, each profession has its own angle, point of view and approach, which always depend on the client's needs, motivation and willingness. Psychological care complements social and spiritual care.

In the early stages of palliative care, "classic" outpatient psychotherapy with 20 or more sessions may be individually appropriate. However, the further a disease progresses towards the terminal and end of life stage, the more the need arises for different types of support and intervention. Psychologists working in palliative care often do not know if there will be a second chance to consult with the client alone, or with the client's loved ones, depending on how fast the disease progresses. Situations and state of health may change rapidly. Those close to the patient may also need support themselves, independent from the patient. Palliative care needs a team of carers who remain in close contact with each other and share knowledge and information relevant to care. Consequently, it is essential for psychologists to be part of a team independent of the care setting. The role of psychologists in palliative care and the competence they need differ in many ways from those necessary in psychiatry or psychotherapy (Sektion Psychologie der DGP 2016; Kasl-Godley/King/Quill 2014).

Task, Roles and Functions of Psychologists

The psychology section of the German palliative care association *"Deutsche Gesellschaft für Palliativmedizin"* has published a job profile for psychologists in palliative care based on current scientific publications (Sektion Psychologie der DGP 2016). The WHO definition of palliative care presents a view of the patient, those close to the patient, and the professional carers as part of a system and subsystems. Therefore, psychological support of patients and those close to them requires an understanding of systemic theories and, consequently, also of systemic interventions. Apart from patients and those close to them, a multi-professional team may also benefit from psychological support and knowledge about complex psychodynamic relationships and complex situations in communication. Psychologists are also experts on psycho-hygiene and self-care and, apart from being experts on scientific statistics, are also able to contribute to scientific research in the field of palliative care.

Of course, trained psychologists that work in palliative care must assume the role of either clinical psychologist or psychotherapist. But they may also lend support in the form of knowledge mediator, lecturer, coach, researcher, counselor for a team and/or an organization, expert on reflection, contemplation and communication, and provide guidance in change processes.

The psychological support of patients/clients and those close to them is not so much focused on the treatment of pathological psychiatric disorders, but rather concentrates on their needs and resources to support their ability to cope, and their well-being. This support encompasses:
- psychological diagnostics: the necessary minimum
- the prevention of psychiatrically relevant disorders
- the reduction of anxiety, depression, demoralization and distress, or at least a change in quality so that it becomes more bearable
- clinical counseling
- crisis intervention
- support in effective, useful and helpful communication
- support in decision-making
- alleviation and/or relief and/or reduction of stressful somatic symptoms with partly psychogenic causes

Issues in Psychological Support

In addition to depression, grief, desperation, fear, anxiety, insecurity and isolation, financial problems and spiritual crisis, there may also be other issues involved in the psychological support of patients. They have to cope with the loss of autonomy, meaning in life, dignity, self-esteem, control, hope or intimacy. Embitterment and demoralization may combine with a sense of helplessness in coping with changes in life and the actual situation. There may be distress due to changes in body image, or concentration disorders, sleep disorders, mood changes and/or mood swings, feelings of shame or guilt, and somatic symptoms. Patients may suffer from social withdrawal, stress, and conflicts in the family, the need to settle urgent matters, unfulfilled sexual desires and needs resulting from a loss of intimacy, and very often from feeling guilty about being a burden to others. There may be issues a patient cannot actually talk to a close person about, like a desire for reconciliation or a dying wish. Looking back on life may be connected with a desire for repentance or finding inner peace or inner freedom (Mehnert/Vehling 2018, 30f.; Kasl-Godley/King/Quills 2014, 366; Sektion Psychologie der DGP 2016).

Issues faced by those close to the patient differ, due to their position and point of view. Being the carer, but also being affected and concerned, may cause distress and difficulties in coping. Distress may also arise from the challenges of organizing daily life and all the demands they may have to face, as well as from fear concerning their own future. A dilemma often faced by those close to the patient is not wanting to be left alone, and yet not wanting the loved one to suffer. The anticipated loss causes grief and bereavement and may lead to a complicated grief or prolonged grief disorder. People closely connected to severely ill patients may also tend to withdraw socially and overstretch themselves to the extent of a complete breakdown (Mehnert/Vehling 2018, 30f.; Kasl-Godley/King/Quills 2014, 366; Sektion Psychologie der DGP 2016). It is important to be aware that distress and anxiety of patients and those close to them may increase reciprocally.

Examples of Interventions

The basis for all interventions is a systemic approach with the aim of supporting and strengthening the system(s) and each person involved individually. Psychological care may also contribute to an interpersonal encounter between patient and psychologist/therapist, in which a sense of connectedness can be re-established. Psychologists sustain people who often cannot endure their own situation. The concept of salutogenesis established by A. Antonovsky (Antonovsky 1979) offers a simple, but clear, theoretical basis for many psychological interventions in palliative care: To achieve a sense of coherence through comprehensibility, manageability and meaningfulness, it is necessary to offer support in understanding, finding meaning in and coping with new and difficult situations, in which life-threatening illness and loss of the loved one have to be faced.

Some psychotherapeutic directions provide rich possibilities for interventions psychologists and psychotherapists can use in palliative care, for example:
– ACT – Acceptance and Commitment Therapy (Sonntag 2017, 71-85),
– hypnotherapy (Schulze/Revenstorf 2017, 155-173),
– existential analysis or existential psychotherapy (Noyon/Heidenreich 2017, 121-135),
– analytical psychology (Dorst 2017, 87-105) or
– mindfulness-based approaches (Heidenreich, Riedel, Michalak 2017, 53-69).
Especially created for use in palliative care are:
– Meaning-centered psychotherapy (Breitbart et al. 2012, 1304-1309),
– CALM (Hales/Lo/Rodin 2010),
– Dignity therapy (Chochinov 2017),
– Schedule for Meaning in Life Evaluation (SMiLE) (Fegg et al. 2008) and
– mindfulness-based supportive therapy (Beng et al. 2013, 144-160).
Three of these psychotherapeutic interventions, CALM, Dignity therapy and SMiLE, are briefly introduced here to provide a general description of what they entail.
a)   CALM, i.e. Managing Cancer and Living Meaningfully (Hales/Lo/Rodin 2010; Mehnert/ Vehling 2018, 33) is a semi-structured individual intervention with four content domains:
   a.   symptom management and communication with healthcare providers
   b.   changes in self and relations with those close
   c.   sense of meaning and purpose
   d.   the future and mortality
   The therapy is a "safe place" to explore fears, to be seen in human terms and to face the challenges of advancing disease. Therapy aims to make depressive symptoms and fear of death more bearable and possibly reduce them, while achieving an increase in spiritual well-being.
b)   Dignity therapy (Chochinov 2017) is based on a definition of the dignity of severely ill people resulting from Chochinov's research. The goal is to strengthen perspectives and practices that preserve dignity in order to reduce any negative influences on dignity from illness-related issues and/ or interaction with others.
   It helps bolster the dignity of dying patients and address their suffering and is a therapeutic intervention inviting individuals with life-limiting illnesses to reflect on matters of importance to them. Dignity therapy

gives patients a chance to record the meaningful aspects of their lives and leave something behind that can benefit their loved ones in the future. It consists of a semi-structured interview which gets recorded, transcribed, edited, and returned to the patient.

c)   The Schedule for Meaning in Life Evaluation (SMiLE) (Fegg et al. 2008) was developed to measure accurately the meaning of life of patients by identifying all areas of life which subjectively give meaning to life, rating the patient's actual level of satisfaction with these areas, and the level of importance assigned to these areas. This instrument helps patients to consciously contemplate their own individual meaningful aspects of life. It also provides a basis for further interventions to strengthen personal resources and coherence. SMiLE also gets used in scientific research to measure the effect of psychological interventions.

Conclusion

Psychologists and psychotherapists in palliative care (in German: *Palliativ-psychologen*) work with their own professional approach, although the topics they discuss with clients can overlap with those relevant to other professions involved. Psychotherapeutic interventions can reduce distress and anxiety and contribute to psychological growth. Psychologists can support teams and staff working in palliative care. Several psychotherapeutic interventions have been developed for patients with advanced life-threatening diseases and their relatives. Since 2013, there has been a curriculum for psychologists in palliative care with a DGP-certificate in Germany, which marks important progress in quality enhancement and assurance (Sektion Psychologie der DGP 2013). Although psychologists do not necessarily belong to the "core" of caregivers, there is still a long way to go in providing all patients in palliative care with the possibility of receiving psychological support in all care settings.

Bibliography

Antonovsky, Aaron (1979): Health, stress, and coping, San Francisco: Jossey Bass.
Beng, Tan S./Chin, Loh E./Guan, Ng C./Yee, Anne/Wu, Cathie/Jane, Lim E. (2013): Mindfulness-based supportive therapy (MBST): proposing a palliative psycho-therapy from a conceptual perspective to address suffering in palliative care, in: American journal of hospice and palliative medicine 32, 2:144-160.

Breitbart, William/Poppito, Shannon/Rosenfeld, Barry/Vickers, Andrew J./Li, Yuelin/ Abbey, Jennifer/Olden, Megan/Pessin, Hayley/Lichtenthal, Wendy/Sjoberg, Daniel/ Cassileth, Barrie R. (2012): Pilot randomized controlled trial of individual meaning-centered psychotherapy for patients with advanced cancer, in: Journal of clinical oncology 30, 12:1304-1309.

Chochinov, Harvey M. (2017): Würdezentrierte Therapie. Was bleibt – Erinnerungen am Ende des Lebens, Göttingen: Vandenhoek und Ruprecht.

Dost, Brigitte (2017): Analytische Psychologie. "Den Tod als Ziel sehen" (C. G. Jung), in: D. Berthold/J. Gramm/M. Gaspar/U. Sibelius (Eds.), Psychotherapeutische Perspektiven am Lebensende. Göttingen: Vandenhoek and Ruprecht, 87-105.

Fegg, Martin J./Kramer, Mechthild/Stiefel, Friedrich/Borasio, Gian D. (2008): Lebenssinn trotz unheilbarer Erkrankung? Die Entwicklung des Schedule for Meaning in Life Evaluation (SMiLE), in: Zeitschrift für Palliativmedizin 9, 4: 238-245.

Gramm, Jan/Münch, Urs (2017), Psychologie und Psychotherapie in der bundes-deutschen Palliativversorgung, in: D. Berthold/J. Gramm/M. Gaspar/U. Sibelius (Eds.), Psychotherapeutische Perspektiven am Lebensende. Göttingen, Vandenhoek and Ruprecht, 33-39.

Hales, Sarah/Lo, Chris/Rodin, Gary (2010): Managing Cancer and Living Meaningfully (CALM) – treatment manual: an individual psychotherapy for patients with advanced cancer. Department of Psychosocial Oncology and Palliative Care, Toronto: Princess Margaret University Health Network.

Heidenreich, Thomas/Riedel, Annette/Michalak, Johannes (2017): Achtsamkeitsbasierte Ansätze: Im Hier und Jetzt (auch) in der letzten Lebensphase, in: D. Berthold/ J. Gramm/M. Gaspar/U. Sibelius (Eds.), Psychotherapeutische Perspektiven am Lebensende. Göttingen, Vandenhoek and Ruprecht: 53-69.

Kasl-Godley, Julia E./King, Deborah A./Quill, Timothy E. (2014): Opportunities for Psychologists in Palliative Care. Working with Patients and Families across the Disease Continuum, in: American Psychologist 69, 4, 364-376.

Mehnert, Anja/Vehling, Sigrun (2018): Psychoonkologische Unterstützung von Patienten und Angehörigen in der Terminalphase, in: FORUM 33, 30-34.

Münch, Urs/Gramm, Jan/Berthold, Daniel (2016): Mehr als Psychotherapie. Psychologisches Arbeiten in Palliative Care, in: Psychotherapie im Dialog 1: 81-85.

Noyon, Alexander/Heidenreich, Thomas (2017): Existentielle Ansätze. Ein Plädoyer für Realitätsorientierung und Menschlichsein, in: D. Berthold/J. Gramm/M. Gaspar/ U. Sibelius (Eds.), Psychotherapeutische Perspektiven am Lebensende. Göttingen: Vandenhoek and Ruprecht, 121-135.

Schulze, Wolfgang/Revenstorf, Dirk (2017): Hypnotherapie. Veränderungsprozesse anstoßen durch Trance, in: D. Berthold/J. Gramm/M. Gaspar/U. Sibelius (Eds.), Psychotherapeutische Perspektiven am Lebensende. Göttingen: Vandenhoek and Ruprecht, 155-173.

Sektion Psychologie der DGP (2013): Basiscurriculum Palliative Care für Psychologen. Reihe Palliative Care Band 5, Bonn: PalliaMed Verlag.

Sektion Psychologie der DGP (2016): Palliativpsychologie – Berufsbild für Psychologinnen und Psychologen in Palliative Care. Online: https://www.dgpalliativmedizin.de/images/Berufsbild_PalliativpsychologIn_DGP_2016.pdf (last access 03/26/2019).

Sonntag, Rainer F. (2017): Akzeptanz- und Commitment-Therapie: Akzeptanz und Engagement bis zuletzt, in: D. Berthold/J. Gramm/M. Gaspar/U. Sibelius (Eds.), Psychotherapeutische Perspektiven am Lebensende. Göttingen: Vandenhoek and Ruprecht, 71-85.

Professionalizing Clinical Ethics Consultation

Training to Encounter Human Suffering via the Assessing Clinical Ethics Skills Tool

Katherine Wasson

Background

The field of clinical ethics consultation emerged in the United States (U.S.) during the late 1970s and early 80s in response to advances in medical technologies that raised ethical questions, specifically in relation to decisions about prolonging life with the assistance of mechanical ventilators and artificial nutrition and hydration. Physicians sought help in understanding and analyzing morally acceptable choices about life and death when using these new technologies. Physicians looked to people with training outside of medicine for different approaches and perspectives on such quandaries. Historically, those who do clinical ethics consultations come from a variety of disciplines including philosophy, theology, chaplaincy, law, social work, medicine, nursing and others. While a relatively small number of individuals now have undergraduate or graduate degrees in bioethics, others gained practical experience through fellowships, internships, shadowing colleagues, or short intensive courses, and others may have no formal training. The variety of pathways to clinical ethics consultation work raises questions about what constitutes the appropriate or sufficient education and training needed in order to respond to patients, their families, and health care teams.

The role of a clinical ethics consultant (CEC) is multi-faceted and key components include identifying and clarifying ethical issues in a case as well as facilitating conversation about value-laden ethical issues in healthcare and, hopefully, reaching an ethically justifiable decision that is agreed by the different parties involved (ASBH 2011). CECs are typically called into a case when there is an implicit or explicit conflict or disagreement about the ethically appropriate options and ways forward in a patient's care. Such cases regularly emerge from an Intensive Care Unit (ICU) and, often, though by no means exclusively, arise regarding disagreements at the end of life (DuVal et al. 2001, Johnson et al. 2012, Moeller et al. 2012, Streuli et al. 2014, Swetz et al. 2007, Tapper et al. 2010, Wasson et al. 2016b). In each case suffering is present, whether physical, emotional, psychological, or spiritual.

Case Study

Mr. Jones is a 67 year-old man who has been in the Medical ICU with Chronic Obstructive Pulmonary Disease (COPD), heart failure, and sepsis for the past 10 days. During the past two days he also developed kidney failure. He is now dying. Mr. Jones has been in the ICU before with pneumonia and eventually returned home. His family, including his wife and two adult sons, visit regularly. His wife is there daily and rarely leaves his room. The sons visit on the evenings and weekends. The family has not yet accepted that Mr. Jones is dying and wants all aggressive interventions to continue, while the healthcare team views these efforts as "futile" because they are not going to enable him to recover and leave the hospital this time. The healthcare team recognizes that multiple organ systems are failing and that even with all the support of the Medical ICU, Mr. Jones is dying. The family thinks the team is "giving up" and claims they are "uncaring," and the team views the family as being "difficult" or "challenging" because they continue to press for the highest level of interventions possible, including attempted resuscitation if he goes into cardiac arrest. Multiple family meetings have been held and both groups are frustrated.

There are multiple ethical issues present in this case, including discovering the patient's wishes if known, respecting his autonomy and choices if possible, identifying the appropriate surrogate decision-maker if Mr. Jones is unable to express his wishes and there is no written documentation of them, and weighing the benefits against the burdens of the interventions. A discussion of these ethical issues with the healthcare team and family will lead to a broader discussion of the goals of care, specifically a shift from a curative to palliative or comfort care approach and weighing of quality vs. quantity of life. Each ethical issue requires knowledge and interpersonal skills to facilitate a sensitive discussion around such issues, highlighting the need to train CECs in this area. Yet, few training tools are available.

Training to Face the Reality of Suffering in Ethics Consultation

In the midst of the disagreement and conflict, there is suffering present for all parties on some level. Mr. Jones is experiencing the burden of his disease and failing organ systems and may be suffering physically from the interventions, e.g. intubation, blood draws, artificial nutrition, or the weight of those interventions. The family is suffering emotionally and psychologically as they watch the patient in this condition. They are also suffering spiritually in the face of the loss of their loved-one. The healthcare team may experience emotional and psychological suffering because they wanted to cure the patient, or at least help him recover and return home, and that goal is not possible. The team may also view the burdens of the ineffective treatments as causing suffering for the patient and be distressed by this situation. Unless the patient has a "Do Not Resuscitate Order" (DNR), the team may also be anxious that they will need to code the patient, which means inflicting harm from the chest compressions, possibly breaking his ribs, while knowing these efforts are highly unlikely to benefit Mr. Jones in the short or long-term. All parties are experiencing suffering on some level and encountering the suffering of others, most acutely the patient's. CECs face human suffering regularly and need to be prepared and competent to deal with this reality, which includes having relevant interpersonal skills. Yet, there are few specific tools available to instruct individuals on what constitutes an ethics consultation, or train them in how to provide a competent ethics consultation.

The Assessing Clinical Ethics Skills (ACES) Project

Unlike chaplains, physicians, and nurses, CECs in the U.S. currently do not have to be certified in order to conduct ethics consultations (The Joint Commission 1992)[1]. While this situation is changing, the content of what constitutes sufficient training for CECs and how to assess their training and skills remains an ongoing debate (Fins et al. 2013, Pearlman et al. 2016, Wasson et al. 2016b). In an attempt to provide some standardization to the field, the American Society for Bioethics and Humanities (ASBH) published the *Core Competencies for Healthcare Ethics Consultation* (ASBH 1998/2011) detailing the knowledge and skills required. In 2018, the ASBH decided to move forward with a certification process via a multiple choice examination and grant successful candidates the status of Healthcare Ethics Consultant-Certified (HEC-C). This examination assesses knowledge and its application in different domains relevant to clinical ethics work, but does not evaluate the interpersonal skills of CECs. While the intellectual content is vital to facilitating ethics consults, the practical, interpersonal skills are equally important when addressing sensitive ethical decisions in contexts where human suffering is present.

In response to this need for training and evaluating the interpersonal skills of CECs, the Assessing Clinical Ethics Skills (ACES) tool was developed at Loyola University Chicago. Four bioethicists with expertise in clinical ethics

---

1   The Joint Commission on the Accreditation of Healthcare Organizations requires hospitals to have access to ethics services, but does not specify what those services should be.

consultation selected the content of the ACES tool based on the ASBH Core Competencies and the Veterans Affairs IntegratedEthics® Program's Ethics Consultant Proficiency Assessment Tool (ECPAT) (Wasson et al. 2016b, US Department of Veterans Affairs 2014). Once the twelve core skills were agreed upon, these clinical ethics experts articulated specific behaviors which the CEC would need to demonstrate for each item and which could be evaluated when observed (see Table 1). For example, Item 1 is *Manage the Formal Meeting.* The specific skills to be evaluated are: *Identify yourself and your role as the ethics consultant; Have each party introduce themselves; Explain the purpose of the consult.*

The ACES tool aims to evaluate the interpersonal skills of CECs and students or trainees in ethics consultation in an educational setting, i.e. during a simulated ethics case consultation. The trainee is given an ethics consultation case and required to perform as a CEC with physicians, nurses, and actors playing the family member(s) or patient in the ethics consultation. The case is video-taped and evaluated in real time by a trained rater watching a live stream from the simulation room. After the simulated consult, the trainee is given feedback on his/her performance in relation to the skills on the ACES tool. The trainee also receives a video recording of his/her performance and, if part of a graduate course, is required to evaluate him/herself using the ACES tool. This format provides multiple opportunities for structured feedback and assessment for the trainee.

Because of the paucity of training tools for ethics consultation and the importance of evaluating the skills of CECs, the authors of the ACES tool developed a website to allow users to access the ACES tool at no charge (https://hsd.luc.edu/bioethics/ethicsconsultskills/). Users wanting to learn about ethics consultation can request access to the website, which includes multiple video-taped ethics consultations designed to demonstrate the various skills a CEC requires to conduct an ethics consultation sufficiently. For each case, the user reviews the instructions on how to score each item on the ACES tool and then views the four scenes of the case. He/she decides whether the CEC in the video should receive a *Done, Not Done,* or *Done Incorrectly* for each item in that scene and submits those answers. Then, the user receives video and written feedback on how his/her answers align with the correct responses. At the end of the case, the user can print out a full report of his/her answers and the correct responses for that case. In addition, the ACES cases are included in *An Ethics Casebook for Hospitals: Practical Approaches to Everyday Ethics Consultations* (Kuczewski et al. 2018). These "skill builder" cases, along with other cases, are set out in the text with descriptions and points of view from stakeholders that enable readers to role-play and analyze the cases themselves or with other CECs.

The aim of the website is to train users to recognize competency and incompetency in the skills of the CECs in the video cases. Making it web-based provides access around the world. Knowing what skills are required to facilitate an ethics consultation is a necessary first step, and these are articulated in the ACES tool. Learning to identify whether the item is *Done, Not Done*, or *Done Incorrectly* by the CEC takes practice and an alignment with the expert raters who designed the tool. The aim of this training is that a user of the website will not only learn to recognize competency and incompetency in the videos, but also begin to apply those standards to his/her own practice (Wasson et al., 2019). This relationship needs to be tested in practice.

Practical Application of the ACES Tool

How does the ACES tool help a CEC work through a consultation? Examining how the tool provides a structure for addressing suffering offers one example. There are multiple items on the ACES tool that have the potential to address different types of suffering during the ethics consultation.

Physical suffering of the patient: The details of the patient's condition will be elicited through *Item 2: Gather the Relevant Data*. Here, the CEC needs to elicit the relevant medical facts, which may include physical discomfort, pain, and uncontrolled symptoms. Finding approaches to address pain and other symptoms should be offered by the healthcare team. If these areas are not addressed, the CEC may need to suggest the involvement of other specialists, such as a palliative care team (if appropriate). This discussion may also be covered in *Item 10: Distinguish ethical dimensions of the consultation from other, often overlapping, dimensions*, which includes the sub-item of *Offer other appropriate ancillary services*.

Emotional, psychological or spiritual suffering: These types of suffering can and should be explored and addressed through multiple items on the ACES tool. The first is *Item 4: Listen well, and communicate interest, respect, support, and empathy to participants* that includes the sub-item, *Express a supportive statement early in the consult*. Recognizing and naming the stress, strain and struggle of those involved in the case is an important way to demonstrate empathy. It can also help the CEC establish rapport with the participants through acknowledging their suffering. *Item 6: Enable participants to communicate effectively and be heard by others*, can be a powerful means of acknowledging suffering and allowing someone to articulate how it is affecting them. *Item 9: Mediate among competing views*, is related to Item 6 and ensures the CEC is facilitating the conversation in a manner that allows all parties to express their views, values, expectations and priorities. Without this item, some participants may dominate the conversation and others may remain largely silent in their suffering. Creating space for all participants to contribute to the conversation can also provide key insights into the patient's wishes and preferences along with helping the CEC identify the ethical dilemmas present.

In addition, *Item 8: Educate participants regarding the ethical dimensions of the case*, includes a number of sub-items that provide opportunities to address suffering. The CEC should identify and articulate what the ethical issues are. This step can be helpful in giving concrete language to the unease surrounding a case. Item 8 requires the CEC not only to identify the ethical issues but also the range of ethically (in)appropriate options as well as explain why these options are justifiable or not. Articulating why this case poses ethical dilemmas and noting where the different values may or do conflict helps the parties clarify their views and may help identify areas of agreement or common ground. It also can assist in the decision-making process as the parties are clearer about what needs to be decided and the basis on which those decisions are made, e.g. clinical considerations vs. quality of life judgements.

Finally, *Item 10* again provides a context in which to address suffering via the sub-item of *Offer other appropriate ancillary services*, which can include other medical consultations, such as palliative care, psychological support, social work, chaplaincy or others. These support services can be for the patient directly or the family members and can address suffering on all levels.

There is a paucity of training mechanisms for CECs, particularly regarding the interpersonal skills needed to facilitate an ethics consultation. Appropriately demonstrating each of the skills identified on the ACES tool is necessary for a CEC to be competent. Making the tool available via the internet allows access globally. Having a means of being trained to recognize competency in the CECs in the cases on the website is one phase of training. Using the ACES tool to evaluate CECs in real time is a second stage needed to train and equip them to address the ethical issues and be attentive to the suffering that is present in ethics consults and have the appropriate skills to facilitate the consult in a way which, hopefully, brings about resolution for all parties.

Acknowledgement: I would like to thank my colleagues, Mark Kuczewski, Kayhan Parsi and Michael McCarthy for their joint work in creating the ACES tool.

Table 17.1   ACES tool items
(© *2016 Loyola University Chicago. Used with permission. All rights reserved*)

Manage the Formal Meeting

1. Identify yourself and your role as the ethics consultant

2. Have each party introduce themselves

3. Explain the purpose of the consult

Gather the Relevant Data

4. Elicit the relevant medical facts in the case

5. Confirm the appropriate decision maker

6. Clarify when needed

Express and Stay within the Limits of the Ethics Consultant's Role During Meetings or Encounters

7. Health professionals and administrators should distinguish their clinical roles from their ethics role as needed

8. Correct errant expectations of participants as needed

Listen Well, and Communicate Interest, Respect, and Empathy to Participants

9. Maintain eye contact

10. Use engaged body language

11. Express supportive statements early in the consult

12. Avoid distracting behaviors

Elicit the Moral Views of the Participants in a Non-Threatening Way

13. Establish the moral views and/or values of participants

14. Establish the wishes and/or expectations of participants

15. Clarify when needed

Enable Participants to Communicate Effectively and Be Heard by Other Participants

16. Give each participant an opportunity to share his or her views

17. Ask clarifying questions

18. Redirect conversation when needed

Accurately and Respectively Represent the Views of Participants to Others

19. Summarize the conversation reflecting back the views of each party

20. Allow participants to confirm or clarify

Educate Participants Regarding the Ethical Dimensions of the Case

21. Identify the ethical issues

22. Identify the range of ethically (in)appropriate options

23. Explain the rationale for the ethically (in)appropriate options

24. Use plain/simple language

Mediate Among Competing Moral Views

25. Identify common goals including areas of agreement

26. Identify areas of disagreement

27. Elicit or propose potential compromise options

Distinguish Ethical Dimensions of the Consultation from Other, often Overlapping, Dimensions

28. Identify relevant legal issues

29. Offer other appropriate ancillary services

Identify and Explain a Range of Ethically Justifiable Options and Their Consequences

30. Summarize potential options/choices already discussed

31. Facilitate discussion about options (pros/cons) including ways forward

Bibliography

American Society for Bioethics and Humanities (1998): Core competencies for health care ethics consultants, Glenview/IL: ASBH.

American Society for Bioethics and Humanities (2011): Core competencies for health care ethics consultants, 2nd edition, Glenview/IL: ASBH.

American Society for Bioethics and Humanities (ASBH) Certification Commission (2018). Online: http://asbh.org/professional-development/certification/hcec-certi-fication-commission (last access 04/01/2019).

DuVal, Gordon/Sartorius, Leah/Clarridge, Brian/Gensler, Gary/Danis, Marion (2001): What triggers requests for ethics consultations? In: Journal of Medical Ethics 27, 1: i24-i29. Online: 10.1136/jme.27.suppl_1.i24 (last access 04/01/2019).

Johnson, Laura S./Lesandrini, Jason/Rozycki, Grace S. (2012): Use of the medical ethics consultation service in a busy Level I trauma center: impact on decision-making and patient care, in: American Surgeon 78, 7:735-740.

Joint Commission on the Accreditation of Healthcare Organizations (1992): Comprehensive Accreditation Manual for Hospitals, Standard Rl.l.l.6.1, at I, The Joint Commission 1992.

Kodish, Eric/Fins, Joseph J./Braddock, Clarence/Cohn, Felicia/Dubler, Nancy N./ Danis, Marion/Derse, Arthur R./Pearlman, Robert A./Smith, Martin/Tarzian, Anita/ Youngner, Stuart/Kuczewski, Mark G. (2013): Quality attestation for clinical ethics consultants: A two-step model from the American Society for Bioethics and Humanities, in: Hastings Center Report 43, 5: 26-36. Online: https://doi.org/10.1002/hast.198 (last access 04/01/2019).

Kuczewski, Mark G./Pinkus, Rosa Lynn/Wasson, Katherine (2018): An ethics casebook for hospitals: Practical approaches to everyday ethics consultations, vol. 2, Washington/D.C.: Georgetown University Press.

Moeller, Jessica R./Albanese, Teresa H./Garchar, Kimberly/Aultman, Julie M./Radwany, Steven/Frate, Dean (2012): Functions and outcomes of a clinical medical ethics committee: a review of 100 consults, in: HEC Forum 24, 2:99-114. Online: 10.1007/s10730-011-9170-9 (last access 04/01/2019).

Pearlman, Robert A./Foglia, Mary Beth/Fox, Ellen/Cohan, Jennifer H./Chanko, Barbara L./Berkowitz, Kenneth A. (2016): Ethics consultation quality assessment tool: A novel methods for assessing the quality of ethics case consultations based on written records, in: The American Journal of Bioethics 16, 3: 3-14. Online: https://doi.org/10.1080/15265161.2015.1134704 (last access 04/01/2019).

Streuli, Jürg C./Staubli, Georg/Pfändler-Poletti, Marlis/Baumann-Hölzle, Ruth/Ersch, Jörg (2014): Five-year experience of clinical ethics consultations in a pediatric teaching hospital, in: European Journal of Pediatrics 173, 5: 629-636. Online: 10.1007/s00431-013-2221-2 (last access 04/01/2019).

Swetz, Keith M./Crowley, Mary Eliot/Hook, C. Christopher/Mueller, Paul S. (2007): Report of 255 clinical ethics consultations and review of the literature, in: Mayo Clinical Proceedings 82, 6:686-691. Online: https://doi.org/10.4065/82.6.686 (last access 04/01/2019).

Tapper, Elliot B./Vercler, Christian J./Cruze, Deborah/Sexson, William (2010): Ethics consultation at a large urban public teaching hospital, in: Mayo Clinic Proceedings 85, 5: 433-38. Online: https://doi.org/10.4065/mcp.2009.0324 (last access 04/01/2019).

U.S. Department of Veterans Affairs/National Center for Ethics in Health Care (2014): Ethics consultant proficiency assessment tool. Online: https://www.ethics.va.gov/ECPAT.pdf (last access 04/01/2019).

Wasson, Katherine/Adams, William H./Berkowitz, Kenneth/Danis, Marion/Derse, Arthur R./Kuczewski, Mark G./McCarthy, Michael/Parsi, Kayhan/Tarzian, Anita (2019): What is the minimal competency for a clinical ethics consult simulation? Setting a standard for use of the Assessing Clinical Ethics Skills (ACES) tool, in: The American Journal of Bioethics Empirical Research 10, 3: 164-172.

Wasson, Katherine/Anderson, Emily/Hagstrom, Erika/McCarthy, Michael/Parsi, Kayhan/Kuczewski, Mark (2016a): What ethical issues really arise in practice at an academic medical center? A quantitative and qualitative analysis of clinical ethics consultations from 2008 to 2013, in: HEC Forum 28, 3: 217-228. Online: DOI: 10.1007/s10730-015-9293-5 (last access 09/13/2021).

Wasson, Katherine/Parsi, Kayhan/McCarthy, Michael/Siddall, Viva Jo/Kuczewski, Mark (2016b): Developing an evaluation tool for assessing clinical ethics consultation skills in simulation based education: The ACES project, in: HEC Forum 28, 2: 103-13. Online: DOI: 10.1007/s10730-015-9276-6 (last access 09/13/2021).

Contributors

PROF. DR. CLAUDIA BOZZARO
is head of the Medical Ethics Division at the Institute of Experimental Medicine at Kiel University.

PROF. DR. MICHAEL COORS
is Associate Professor of Theological Ethics and head of the Institute of Social Ethics at University of Zurich.

DR. TOBIAS EICHINGER
is Senior Teaching and Research Assistant at the Institute of Biomedical Ethics and History of Medicine at the University of Zurich.

DR. TUBA ERKOC BAYDAR
is Assistant Professor at Ibn Haldun University, Istanbul.

TARA FLANAGAN, PHD
is Assistant Professor of Theology and Religious Studies at Maria College and chaplain at New York-Presbyterian/Jansen Hospice and Palliative Care.

PROF. DR. OTTMAR FUCHS
is Professor Emeritus of Practical Theology at the Faculty of Catholic Theology at the University of Tübingen.

PROF. DR. HILLE HAKER
is Professor for Theological Ethics and holds the Richard McCormick SJ Chair of Catholic Moral Theology at Loyola University Chicago.

PROF. DR. ILHAN ILKILIC, MD, PHD
is Chair and Professor at the Department of History of Medicine and Ethics at the Istanbul University Faculty of Medicine and director of the Institute for Health Sciences of Istanbul University.

REV. JÜRGEN JANIK
is head of the catholic hospital chaplaincy at the University Medical Center Mainz.

PROF. DR. CARLO LEGET
is Professor of Care Ethics at the University of Humanistic Studies in Utrecht and Endowed Professor of Ethics and Spirituality in Palliative Care at the same university.

DR. BERND OLIVER MAIER
is vice President of the German Association for Palliative Medicine and head Physician of Palliative Medicine and Interdisciplinary Oncology at the St. Josefs-Hospital in Wiesbaden.

PROF. DR. CHRISTOF MANDRY
is Professor of Moral Theology and Christian Social Ethics at the Department of Catholic Theology, Goethe University Frankfurt.

MICHAEL MCCARTHY, PHD
is Associate Professor at the Neiswanger Institute for Bioethics and Health Policy at Loyola University Chicago Stritch School of Medicine.

DYPL. PSYCH. PP URS MÜNCH
works as psycho-oncologist and part of the Palliative Care Team in DRK Kliniken Berlin. He serves as Vice President of the German Association for Palliative Medicine.

PROF. DR. ARNE JOHAN VETLESEN
is Professor of Philosophy at the University of Oslo.

AANA MARIE VIGEN, PHD
is Associate Professor of Christian Social Ethics at Loyola University Chicago.

DR. GWENDOLIN WANDERER
is Scientific Coordinator of the project "Medical Ethics in Clinical Pastoral Care" at the chair of Moral Theology and Social Ethics, Goethe University Frankfurt.

KATHERINE WASSON, PHD
is Associate Professor and bioethicist at the Neiswanger Institute for Bioethics at Loyola University Chicago Stritch School of Medicine.

PROF. DR. KNUT WENZEL
is Professor of Systematic and Fundamental Theology at the Department of Catholic Theology, Goethe University Frankfurt.